# SMART COOKIES DON'T CRUMBLE

### A Modern Woman's Guide to
### Living and Loving Her Own Life

To be a smart cookie, you'll discover how to:

- Unscramble your life and learn how to make the right choices—for you
- Remove the "cloak of inferiority" that keeps you from getting the success you deserve
- Create your own second chances
- Establish stronger, more intimate relationships while maintaining a clear personal identity
- Accept the Sonya Friedman gospel: THE BEST IS YET TO COME!

"I've discovered something true. You have control over three things—what you think, what you say and how you behave. To make a change in your life, you must recognize that these gifts are the most powerful tools you possess in shaping the form of your life. Use them wisely and to the fullest. You can be a smart cookie, starting now."

---

"If you're a smart cookie, you'll buy this book. It's a real eye-opener."
—Mary Ellen Pinkham, author of
*Mary Ellen's Best of Helpful Hints*

---

Sonya Friedman has been host of *Sonya*, a nationally syndicated TV talk show; a columnist for *Ladies' Home Journal;* a practicing psychologist; and author of the national bestseller *Men Are Just Desserts.*

# SMART COOKIES DON'T CRUMBLE

## A Modern Woman's Guide to Living and Loving Her Life

## SONYA FRIEDMAN

POCKET BOOKS

New York   London   Toronto   Sydney   Tokyo   Singapore

POCKET BOOKS, a division of Simon & Schuster
1230 Avenue of the Americas, New York, NY 10020

ISBN: 0-671-69580-0

First Pocket Books printing May 1986

15   14   13   12   11   10   9   8   7   6

POCKET and colophon are registered trademarks of
Simon & Schuster.

Printed in the U.S.A.

To the women who have shaped my life—

My mother, who never really lived her life but by allowing me to observe her existence motivated me to live my own;

My mother-in-law, who was my role model for successfully combining work and family;

My daughter, who has the privilege of choice and a chance to learn from my mistakes;

My friends and clients, who continue to survive their struggles and grow stronger in spite of their wounds;

And to Connie deSwaan, collaborator and friend, whose fluent skills have permitted me to share my message.

# Contents

*After a while you learn the subtle
difference between holding a
hand and chaining a soul,
And you learn that love doesn't
mean leaning and company
doesn't mean security,
And you begin to learn that kisses
aren't contracts and presents
aren't promises,
And you begin to accept your de-
feats with your head up and your
eyes open, with the grace of an
adult, not the grief of a child,
And you learn to build all your
roads on today because tomorrow's ground is too uncertain
for plans.
After a while you learn that even
sunshine burns if you get too
much.
So plant your own garden and decorate your own soul, instead of
waiting for someone to bring you
flowers.
And you learn that you really can
endure . . . that you really are
strong,
And you really do have worth.*

—ANONYMOUS

# SMART COOKIES DON'T CRUMBLE

# Introduction

It was a balmy September evening in Savannah, Georgia—an hour's ride from a friend's summer house. We'd all arrived there the day before for a reunion. Not the classic reacquaintanceship of school chums, but a simple reunion that was more like a ceremony of friendship. Though we spoke frequently by phone, we four women, living in different cities, separated by commitments to professions and relationships, had scarcely seen each other over the years.

The three friends were women I'd met in my adult life, persons to whom I felt a special closeness. They were a kind of extended family for me, women with whom I could be honest and vulnerable, and they with me. Now we were sitting in a restaurant in Savannah, clinking glasses to toast our friendship and to celebrate, in a poignant way, where we'd come from and where we'd gotten to. Each of us remarked that twenty years ago we'd never have predicted that our lives would take the courses they did.

I think these lives, the lives of my friends, are remarkable. We all came from similar backgrounds and had the identical forces exerted upon us: marry as soon as you can, have children, understand that life may be hard, and if it is, what can you do? Three of us married young, believing it was right for us at the time, and loved the men we married. The fourth, putting off marriage until her forties, still struggled to accept what it would mean in her life. We *were* remarkable, all of us. Let me share the reasons why.

I married young and today my marriage is approaching the twenty-eight-year mark. By the age of twenty-six, I had had two children. Thirty was the crisis year for me; was my life over? Legend had it that a woman peaked at thirty; then it was over—whatever "it" was. All I knew was that I needed something beyond my home, a life to carve out for myself in addition to children, husband and hearth. I struggled to reconcile those conflicting feelings in an era when so few women even considered meaningful work, much less careers. My mother-in-law, a practicing dentist, showed me it could be done—that marriage and a career were not irreconcilable. The choice of a career was frightening, but I took my chances and went ahead to see what I could do. I've had a variety of careers—with successes and failures. I wouldn't have it any other way—no regrets!

Claudia, raised by very traditional European parents, was taught to sew, knit, cook, keep house and care for children—skills perfected by her at the age of twelve. Her mother thought she was training her daughter to be a good wife for a better husband; Claudia took those skills with her when she left their home at twenty to live alone. She wanted to be a painter; marriage could wait. Several proposals were turned down. Claudia feared she'd turn into a doting, accommodating wife, asking permission to squeeze lemon into her husband's tea, as her own mother did for her father. She'd been well trained in her early years—that reflexive tending to others was always close to the surface. So she became a woman with a career, surviving lean years with optimism. But she hungered for a family of her own, a child. At forty-two, Claudia married. Now she must come to terms with what that marriage means and the fact that she may or may not be able to have the child she wants.

Paulette—high-spirited, funny, delightful—turned her energies to work after two marriages and two divorces. Then she fell in love, in spite of herself, with a dynamic, successful black man. Her choice was a difficult one for a woman coming from a conservative midwestern background. At forty-five, Paulette found what she wanted in Dan, and she feels exceptional love, fidelity and loyalty for him. She loves the very fact that he is alive, and that he chooses to share his life with her. He feels the same about her. Their relationship is at once calm and intense. And Paulette, once devoted to her career, has taken a sabbatical—giving herself one year at home, working part-time but focusing on their relationship.

Rebecca, talented and warm, was divorced six years ago after twenty years of marriage to her childhood sweetheart. Her husband left her at the age of forty for a much younger woman. By then her three children were teenagers, and motherhood was all she knew. What would happen to her? She had no marketable skills, nor did she know what would please her or how to find it. Native creativity, a few contacts and some good fortune helped guide her—she became a success-ful designer. For a few years she faced singlehood, then met a man she could love; he died tragically. Years later, she met another man, ten years younger than she. Still involved with him, she must confront Frank's feelings: although he loves her, he cannot marry her because he wants a child. At forty-six she cannot give him what he wants, and she's saddened to think of the loss of this man from her life.

## Introduction

Sitting in the restaurant, we four raised our glasses, toasted the future and wondered, what's next? We'd come through so far—we hadn't crumbled during the painful times, the disappointments, the periods of relentless panic. Everything was okay. Each of us anticipated a lot more work ahead to improve our lives for ourselves and others, but we were facing it with optimism, a certain degree of excitement, and a minimum, now, of fear. That night in Savannah I had the keener sense of something I'd always known—*smart cookies don't crumble!* And we four were smart cookies!

What I want to share with you in this book is exactly that: how you can become a smart cookie, too.

Life is full of positive stresses and agonizing shocks, immense pleasures and indescribable pain. Blessings and losses will be with us forever, like the air we breathe. Each life is unique—*your* life is unique—and it deserves the best of attention and careful planning. That means being a smart cookie.

In my years of private practice as a clinical psychologist, I've seen so many women tormented by doubts about themselves. According to them, they "cannot." They cannot resolve conflicts about their marriages, they cannot get a job. They cannot leave an abusive, alcoholic or childlike husband. They cannot stop crying when they speak to a parent. They cannot manage their children. They cannot see life in terms of anything but limitations drawn up by someone else. They cannot visualize a future without the ever-present chorus of complaints from others. They cannot live and they *can* crumble.

If I'd asked any of them straight out what they were most fearful of, most would have said, "making a decision." I understand this. I've been there too, full of doubt but moving forward step by step.

The choices open to you are vast, astonishing, challenging. It takes courage to clarify what you want (and how much of it will satisfy you), to pinpoint a choice and put into operation an abundance of drive, plans and backup systems to get it done.

The world's a lot more complicated now. It spins hundreds of times faster than it did forty years ago, when girls grew up to be nurses, teachers, mothers or maiden aunts. These four permissible choices existed in a fairly predictable society.

Today's standards are high-geared, competitive. Some women feel like misfits because they don't meet the new standards. Others consider themselves failures because they have no aspirations or any interest in accomplishments outside the home.

Feminism created an emotional, political and economic shift that is still resonating. Women can have more—I promise you that—but some are backing off or seriously considering withdrawal into that old, sheltered world, renewing old values about "women's place" in the home.

Betty Friedan analyzed this backlash in her exceptional book *The Second Stage*. Her warning is poignant: "Beware of that return to nostalgia for the simple days when women had no choice. In the fear, and even actual resentment, of the hard choices women face today, beware of the temptation to believe it is even possible, much less desirable, to go back."

Be a smart cookie. Do not go back; do not even stay as you are! Go forward with energy. Go forward knowing that you can reconstruct your life, or at the very least tidy it up so you can enjoy it more. You have a right and a responsibility to enjoy your life, to be excited by it.

The purpose of this book is to help you discover what matters to you and how to sustain it as a positive force in your life. Be a smart cookie. Discover how your true "growth stages" shape your future. You'll see how the first thirty years of life are not the end of youth and opportunities, but in fact are the totality of childhood. The ten years that follow are "middlescence" for you. During middlescence you can find the formula that will start to reshape your life. Smart cookies—and you'll be one—will have a life plan, a map that can be revised with paths that can be rerouted.

In the years from forty to fifty, you'll realize the true beginning of adulthood. It's a time for evaluation, replacement and replenishment. You will take care of unfinished business, explore even greater possibilities and deal with your relationships again. You will learn to live the next thirty or forty years in the best psychological and physical health.

To be a smart cookie, you'll discover how to

• Unscramble your life and learn how to make a choice. How to be guided by ideas on constructing and activating a master plan.

• Remove the "cloak of inferiority" from around your shoulders. You'll learn what's necessary to build self-confidence and start thinking of yourself as a success, not a failure.

• Say no without guilt or fear; to gain personal power by letting others know what you really want.

• Be guided to create a second chance; how to get through the various crises that may be stopping you from moving forward.

• Establish stronger, more intimate relationships while maintaining a clear personal identity.

• Survive divorce, singledom and loss without bitterness or alienation.

• Understand and express your sexuality within and without marriage.

• Accept the gospel: The best is yet to be. You can be reborn every day if you live your life as a smart cookie.

I've discovered something true. You have control over three things—*what you think, what you say* and *how you behave.* To make a change in your life, you must recognize that these gifts are the most powerful tools you possess in shaping the form of your life. Use them wisely and to the fullest. You can be a smart cookie, starting now.

# 1

## Don't Put Your Life on Hold

When she was nineteen, Ann Martell took a bit part in a campus variety show for the fun of it. Her role required that she carry signs across the stage, and that was about it. The part didn't lead to a future in acting, but while on stage she caught the eye of the lead singer in a group called the Mitchell Trio. A year later she wedded him and became the inspiration for a number of his songs. She's Annie Denver—now ex-wife of singer John Denver.

For nearly ten of the sixteen years of their marriage, Annie was basically content to be a wife and mother, but all along—even from the first year—she felt "an edge of unhappiness." Something was missing. "I couldn't define it then," she recalled in a private interview with me, "but eventually I knew I needed a focus outside my marriage. There was only John for me, and he traveled a lot. When we first met, we had a long-distance romance. We'd talk on the phone, then I'd fly out and join him—pretty glamorous and exciting stuff. It's not the same in marriage. That first year was the roughest of my life. John and I married without really knowing each other and suddenly we were struck by the enormous differences between us. But we both wanted a good marriage and worked at it. And it got better."

They'd been married about seven years when they decided to adopt two children. "It was a highlight, a joy, to finally have children," she continued. "And, coincidentally, about that time John became really successful. So there were the children to care for, then a lot of travel and socializing with John. My life was full, but still there was a part of me that was unhappy!"

Annie grew up in a traditional midwestern home in Minnesota. She enrolled in college, not knowing where an education would take her, majoring in art. When she met John in her junior year, she was a rather innocent girl. Their relationship sealed her future. "I just remember being anxious to get married so I wouldn't have to deal with school or make decisions about what to do. There was real security in knowing I'd be married. My parents were for it too, since nothing else was ever expected of me. My parents were wonderful, but happy enough if I got Cs in school. Achievement wasn't important. I was just this sweet little pretty girl. That's all I had to be."

There were times she wasn't happy, but didn't talk about it. "Who would talk to the wife of John Denver about being happy or unhappy?" she asked. "I was married to a well-loved, famous man who wrote songs about me. And he *liked* being married, having a home and children. Then, about six years ago, whatever change was taking place in me started to come out. At first I thought the problems originated with John. I think women tend to feel that way: If only my husband would change . . . if only he would be *that* way, not *this* way. . . .''

As she began to explore the problems in her life, Annie was challenged by a number of questions that had never been asked of her: What do *you* want? What do *you* think? What's really important to you? Simple questions, really, but as Annie told me, "it never occurred to me to look at my life, working from those questions. I thought of my life as a juggling act—and that the juggling was the problem. I was basically like a lot of women; I did what I was told to do."

Annie began to change. "I always thought a marriage had to do with being happy. But in the process of analyzing my situation I was forced to see how relationships can work best. First, you want to be supportive of each other, and second, relationships are about growth and expansion. What it came down to was that our marriage was about my staying the same while John went out to perform, join causes, hungering to grow in his way."

There were painful issues they never discussed, things Annie was willing and not willing to accept in the relationship. "John said to me when I was in therapy for a while, 'You're not the girl I married.' That was the truth, the real truth."

Being married to a celebrity has its benefits and drawbacks. A much-admired performer is adored by fans, pampered, given vast quantities of approval. Often, it's difficult to make a transition to the more basic, nonworshipful home environment. And, for Annie, there were times when she was living a double-standard marriage; she, the dutiful wife at home; he, on the road, not always alone.

On her fifteenth wedding anniversary, Annie broke

the news to John—she could no longer stay in the marriage. "John is who he is and I am who I am. The marriage didn't work anymore. We both gave it a good shot. But basically I ended it because I changed and John changed, but not in compatible ways."

Annie may have started life as the dutiful good girl with no aspirations beyond marriage, but she answered a need, a call to take her life off hold and meet the changes in herself. Annie's enrolled in school now, working toward being a marriage counselor and family therapist. She is optimistic about her future and the possibility of entering a close relationship with a man. "I know it's difficult for women to turn on that little switch in themselves and make decisions that can change things," she concluded. "I feel that most of all it's important to be good to yourself and know that it's okay if you are. You can do anything you set your mind to if you believe things can change."

Annie is brave. She's taken her life off hold, been willing to change what wasn't right for her any longer. When some of us think of change, we shudder at what it may mean. The unknown looms darkly. It need not be so. *To take your life off hold and begin to live more productively, change is an essential factor.*

How do you feel about change?

Try this: You are walking down the street and are stopped by someone you haven't seen in five years. You hear this first: "You've changed."

If you're like most people, these two words will stop you—you're flattered, peeved, amused, curious. Perhaps you'll also experience a mild physical reaction to the comment: an intake of breath, a quickening of the body, a rush of pleasure, a blush.

"You've changed," the speaker has observed, and

you still haven't responded. Your brain is all the while automatically processing bits of information about yourself. For a split second, you don't know precisely what the speaker has in mind about his or her perception of you at the moment.

Perhaps your story is like one of these three:

• Once known as a tranquil soul, you've decided to take a vehement stand against a spouse's (or employer's) inconsiderate behavior. You will no longer be bullied into losing every marital battle, neither will you cower in the presence of a boss. The speaker is right. You've taken your life off hold. *You've changed.*

• In those five years you've been leveled a number of times by disappointments, conflicts. You've taken a few body blows, but you're resilient. It's been a challenge to keep yourself together and you think you have. You've gained a maturity, a sparkle that shows. Your life's off hold. *You've changed.*

• You were once everyone's embodiment of the adjusted single woman. Life absorbed you as you pursued exciting possibilities, kept a watchful eye out for empty promises. You met a man. Marriage, you said on your wedding day, will not turn *me* into a mindless bride, a cipher, "the little woman," a nobody. One year later your friends point out contrasting attitudes between those vows and the way it is now. You've put your life on hold. Even shopping for cough syrup (to remedy *your* cold) is a family affair. Your habit now is to solicit your husband's advice on the merits of one brand over the other—in fact, he's a consultant no matter what the problem. Transformed into a clinger, *you've changed!*

What's the appropriate reply to "you've changed" in these three cases? "In what way?" "What do you mean?" "Thank you!" "No, I haven't really." "So have you." "I'm sorry, that's the way it is."

Each woman's answer will be guided by how she feels about the change, or lack of it, in her life. Is she content with this change or uncomfortable with it? Is she someone who prefers to stay the same and keep her life on hold? Did the change enrich her life? Would she be uncertain about how to respond, how to behave when the speaker indicated anger, mockery, good humor, respect? Might it be easier for her to shrug off the comment than to reveal anything about herself? In contrast, would the question provoke defensiveness or anger? Does the mere thought of change, whether caused by the passage of time, or by a different social status, frighten her?

How we feel about change, in whatever form, helps to illustrate and define how we see ourselves. Some liken change to putting a hand on a hot stove—pull away quickly, reflexively, because it smarts! Blessedly it's over in a wink of an eye before the heat leaves a serious mark. Many believers in the hot-stove theory also think they've "learned" how to avoid being burned by never lighting another stove. Instead, they take their cooler cues about change by constantly checking the calendar, the marketing list, the cupboards, fussing with the creases on the heirloom tablecloth. They find solace in routine, familiarity, replenishment; plans for the future are made on the basis of yesterday's formula.

Continuity and organization are important in keeping us secure. On this I concur. We need to know where we belong, what our lives contain and the time and energy necessary needed to keep our lives going. But if no change is change enough for us, life cannot be fulfilling.

Though our feelings about change are a personal matter, there are some common fears that everyone understands. The idea of change can signify a sense of loss, a fear of the unknown ("Why tempt fate—things may turn out worse!"). It can mean that you feel some power in your grasp but you are afraid that you don't know how to use it ("No one expects me to stand up for myself, and I'm not sure if I know how"). Maybe you are afraid that change will provoke envy in others, that they won't include you any longer in their inner circle ("I won't tell anyone I was given a big raise. They'll think I was making it up to the boss").

Or perhaps you feel that if you change, people who matter to you won't accept and love you when you're "different"—they prefer you the way you are ("Charlie kids me about my weight, but I know he doesn't mind it, really"). Finally, there's a recurrent, all-pervasive fear that as one facet of your life shifts, all other facets will shift along with it until it's unrecognizable. You fear that change could create an uncontrollable ripple effect, with you caught in the eddy. So instead of putting a toe in the water, you keep your life on hold.

Change is something we all resist. And, in resisting it, we may discover that once again we've pushed the button that keeps us on hold—stuck at one level but yearning to step up to another. What is it that keeps us from taking the journey forward or up, and allows movement only from side to side or even, despairingly, in a downward spiral?

The mistaken belief is that most of us are *destined* to stick on hold; that we cannot change. We build the case for not changing based on negative experiences in our lives and on the cumulative effect of self-fulfilling prophecies that begin with others who try to tell us who we are. The cause, we say, is our "gene pools," our temperaments; or we're the products of a neighborhood or region; or we're children of deprivation or privilege and we assume that economics automatically shapes character. "You're never going to amount to much," a mother may repeat to us over and over again. If we don't succeed, it's no surprise to us or to the mother who first made the judgment. And if we don't "amount to much," then it's not our fault: Mother obviously knew something about us that prompted the observation in the first place.

"In most of us," said philosopher William James, "by the age of thirty, the character has set like plaster, and will never soften again." James was satisfied with his indictment of the human personality as immutable. Hard as a rock, though not a rock. I don't think the chemical makeup of plaster has changed much since 1887, when this observation was made, but it seems to me that one does not want to be fixed in plaster. The stuff's quite fragile—droppage means breakage: in which case you change in spite of yourself!

I would agree that there are predictable links between one's history and one's future. We do not arise each day with no memory of who we are and where we've been. However, it is unrealistic and nonsensical to be guided by a theory that sorely limits your chances. In 1887, opportunities were pretty much circumscribed by one's social class, though countless examples can be cited of people who rose from nowhere to somewhere. In 1887, women wore whalebone corsets, were by and large chattel to men, and were not expected to do more than alter their marital status or change frocks for a sail on the lake.

In 1887, a woman's diary held her dreams captive.

Now, nearly one hundred years later, it is *theory* about our limitations that keeps us in bondage. We carry on elaborate conversations in our heads about why we cannot change, or seek agreement from others over oceans of coffee, presenting friends with arguments loaded in favor of staying the same. "You know me, Estelle," you say with a laugh. "Can't keep my spice rack in order—imagine me wanting to open a bakery!"

Do imagine. What does it take to open a bakery? Can this woman learn orderliness, and if she can't, how much would it cost her to hire someone whose specialty it is—after she opens shop! Does she want the bakery, truly, or just the idea of a bakery? *Is she a woman who wants to make a difference in her life or one who is happy to merely talk about making a difference?* Does she really want to take her life off hold?

Consider Jane, who tells me of her disappointments in life, of her dismay at not catching sight of a single dream. Jane loves medicine—it excites her. She's smart and learns quickly. It is a profession that matters to her, but she was not permitted to go to medical school. Her parents discouraged her; it was not a "suitable" profession for a woman, not did they intend to bankroll her. Nursing school was enough.

Now Jane reveals another side of her life. Discouraged from entering medical school and silently lamenting it, she marries the closest thing she can find to a doctor—a nice young man who is studying to be a psychoanalyst. He is fired by ambition and this pleases Jane. He can achieve for her and she can share in his glory.

They are married two years when Ben flunks out of school—the pressure has been too much for him. He takes a low-energy teaching job. Though Jane is frustrated by her life, she learns to ride along with it, making modifications and adjustments as her family grows to include twin sons. Then lightning strikes.

At a family wedding, a successful cousin whom she was very close to when a young girl is moved by Jane's impassioned tale about missing out on medical school. Sipping champagne, Vera suggests an equitable financial arrangement—she will pay for Jane's schooling and will take repayment plus a ridiculously low interest rate when Jane begins practicing. Feeling suddenly like a blind woman given sight, Jane nevertheless controls her excitement over the extraordinary deal, excusing herself from answering directly until she speaks to Ben.

Ben thinks the plan foolish—Jane's too old. Who starts medical school at thirty-four? Who will care for the twins? Who will *he* be if she's a medical school graduate and he's teaching history at a boys' high school?

Jane swallows Ben's reminders of her wifely duties. His scornful response is nothing compared to the emotional tempest boiling inside her. What if she has held up the image of going to medical school as an ideal, then she gets in and it turns out not to matter at all? What if she cannot pass a single course her first semester and fails? Could she deal with being called "doctor"?

Jane is conducting serious debates within herself. Finally, the focus of the conflict becomes displaced and her doubts are projected onto her cousin. How dare Vera throw her weight around? Jane conjectures angrily. So Vera has money—*so what!* The medical school offer was not a gesture of generosity at all, but Vera's way of showing off.

Jane is convinced by these arguments. Fuming, she calls Vera and tells her off, reciting a litany of imagined insults. Why, Jane demands, was Vera rude to her mother? Why did she leave the wedding so early? Why did she have to make everyone feel like paupers by being driven up to the chapel in a limousine? After ten minutes of abusive rage, Jane feels self-righteous. Vindicated. She doesn't need Vera or the stupid offer. She's got her Ben, her twins, her part-time nursing career, her dream of getting into medical school. . . .

And she also has her predicament. Throughout her life, Jane felt deprived. No one had ever before supported her medical school goal. What unfolded when Vera made her surprising offer was an effective, realistic, financially secure chance at honest-to-goodness self-fulfillment; Jane could be a doctor if she so chose. With this offer she would no longer have to bear grudges against unenlightened parents who subscribed to outdated ideas of how good daughters should lead their lives. Nor could a husband with grievances of his own against the "villainous" world out there hold her back.

Jane is trapped between needing to relieve the pain of not getting what she's always wanted and the fear of failing herself and failing others. Part of her dilemma, too, was a fear of success. Turning down a tempting offer wasn't easy. To complicate matters, Jane had to make the transition from feeling good—even joyful—to becoming antagonistic, childish and spiteful toward a possible benefactor. Not many women have the opportunity to reject such bounty as if it were an insult.

What will happen to Jane? She will sustain her pose of a victim of circumstance until she can make peace with her cousin or find another Vera years down the road. The course of her life will depend on whether or not she really wants to make a change, or whether she will be content to simply talk and dream about it for the rest of her days, continuing to bathe in resentment because her life has not given her a break.

# The Traps That Keep Us on Hold

Like Jane, we all have weaknesses—traps—that make us vulnerable and manage to stop us. When the trap is operative, life is switched onto hold indefinitely. To make a difference in your life, and not just *talk* about making a difference, you need to start by identifying the traps that keep you spinning your wheels, getting you nowhere.

Since Jane's story draws our attention to a fear of success and failure, let's start there.

### TRAP #1: A FEAR OF SUCCESS
### AND A FEAR OF FAILURE

"Now that I'm here, where am I?" the talented and doomed singer Janis Joplin, the pearl of the sixties rock generation, said of her success. An exciting performer, Joplin spoke openly about her desire for stardom, her need for the love of her fans and her hometown's respect. We've all had thoughts like these, but here's the twist:

When she achieved her goals ("Now that I'm here") she doubted their meaning and her place in the scheme of things ("Where am I?"). This is the devastating fear that troubles those of you with a fear of success. Countless women share this trap with Joplin, and not just those who are most visible, striving for greatness, celebrity, astounding fortunes, political or social clout or merely their name in the papers.

Included among those with an identifiable fear of success are overweight women who desperately want to lose pounds but sabotage their dieting programs for fear that the physical change will alter their relationships ("My best friend is overweight too, and she'll be jealous and won't like me anymore if I lose weight"). Or the woman who avoids promotion at work because her husband would be threatened by her new high salary.

No matter how you scrutinize success, dissect its significant parts, poke it with a stick to see if you're in imminent danger of a "life-threatening" hug by one of its tendrils, even knock it down so it hits the mat as many times as Rocky I, II or III, success feels good and wears well when you've wanted it, gotten it and liked it. Success can be tough on you because it *will* cost you something, but it is also exciting, generous, full of surprises and plain good fun.

What are the dynamics that keep you from succeeding? What do you think happens that stops you short of success, no matter how much effort you give it? In some cases it's easier going back to what was, or stopping short of what could be, than going full forward! When you drop back, retreat offers cool comfort, where there are no surprises.

For example, the dieter who wants to lose sixty pounds may stop at a forty-five-pound loss, then indulge in a week's worth of anything resembling fudge ripple, thereby adding eight pounds onto the yet-to-be-lost fifteen-pound goal. To succeed, any dieter has to give up calories—what could be simpler? And what could be more difficult for hundreds of thousands of women who face the diet success crisis every day?

Let's backtrack a minute to the idea of "giving up" one thing to get another. It's important here.

My feeling is that life is a balance sheet. *To get, you must give.* There are few pluses without an equal number of minuses. There is no cake without the calories. The executive who puts in a ninety-hour week gives up a more intimate personal life than the forty-hour-a-week laborer, but she gets what she's chosen—her name on the board of directors and the perks and all the problems that come with her position. So what are you willing to sacrifice—time, energy, friendships, money, whatever—to get what you want? When you know what's expected of you, you can make your decision about what you are willing to give up for success and take responsibility for it.

Now suppose that success, as you visualize it in relation to your life, looks and feels remarkably good. However, it's the fear of failure that's dangling above your head on a fine cord. What is the fear of failure?

Look at it this way. While the fear of success can be described more as a fear of the obligations, commitments and strategies involved in reaching a goal, fear of failure touches on other dominant attitudes. When you fear failure, *you fail to act.* Perhaps you feel that by acting you'll prove that you're incompetent, inadequate, not up to standard. There will be hard evidence —a bungled job or relationship. We've seen people like this every day. They're afraid to learn how to drive, apply for a job, go on a blind date, go back to school. This trap is a touchy one, literally, since those with a fear of failure often excuse themselves from acting because they're either too "sensitive" or too "shy." Operate from a fear of failure and you have no choice but to fail to get what you want.

There's not a soul among us who hasn't experienced either a fear of success or a fear of failure. We all know what it means. The question I have for those of you who feel immobilized, trapped here, is: Do you want the fear or the thing you want? Do you want to live your life saying, "If only?"

"Some people spend their lives failing and never notice," says one cynical character in Judith Rossner's novel *Attachments*. Be someone who notices the course of your life. Failure teaches if you let it. You learn to readjust, discard, amend, change direction and grow toward a goal. And when the goal is success, success on your terms, it's always worth your best shot.

## TRAP #2: BE GRATEFUL FOR LITTLE FAVORS

The "little favors" trap is one in which others toss you just enough satisfaction to keep you from seeking a higher goal or trying to change yourself. Let's take a classic example—the woman ignored, wronged and scorned. This story had a violent outcome.

Journalist Ellen Goodman once described the controversial murder of Dr. Hyman Tarnower, the much heralded Scarsdale Diet doctor, by fifty-seven-year-old school headmistress Jean Harris as a case of a woman who'd "learned all too well how to swallow mouthfuls of humiliation in return for tidbits of attention." Sympathize with Mrs. Harris's position and you will understand how tantalizing those tidbits can be to a starving woman. Tidbits kept Jean Harris coming back to the doctor, until the pressure of anger, jealousy and, no doubt, self-loathing, exploded one fateful night and Tarnower fell, shot "accidentally" by this woman who'd loved him for fourteen years.

"Tidbits" of attention, affection or even anger can tempt *any* woman who feels herself at the mercy of the alternative—*nothing*. An interesting but grim conclusion, I think, and a critically faulty judgment. "Nothing" is not a reasonable alternative to the bare minimum, meted out in spiteful doses. If a woman believes that anything is better than nothing, she will shift emotional priorities from getting what she wants (an enriching love association) to settling for whatever is tossed in her direction (minimal acknowledgment of her needs, intermittent sex, a small monthly stipend, or whatever else it may be that binds her to him). Then she is grateful for little favors, as was Jean Harris. Without little favors, she reasons, she is lost.

There are so many women who come to see me with a similar life story summed up by these words: "At least I have a man." They describe a husband's or boyfriend's shortcomings—he's a drinker, a womanizer, a man incapable of keeping a job, a liar or bully, an inadequate father—and then go on to enumerate what's necessary to transform him into a functioning, giving adult. Their plaints are, unfortunately, a measure of how women still value themselves—they believe they are nothing without a man, so they stay, no matter what. The result? A trade-off that keeps them trapped, stuck on hold. Why? They are grateful that they have a roof over their heads, a man's shoes under their beds, "someone to dress up and take out on a Saturday night," as one patient expressed it so vividly about a husband she didn't love.

Let's take another example. You're a secretary (teacher, saleswoman, factory worker) who gets a salary every week, and a certain respect that comes with eight or ten years of seniority. But the company doesn't interest you any longer, you're bored with the routine and the familiarity of the faces on the floor. You feel you haven't any place to aspire to within the organization. You're still there promptly every morning, though, knowing that *at least you've got a job*. It may be the wrong job, but it counts on Fridays when you reach for that paycheck. You're "grateful" for that.

*When you're grateful for little favors, you will always empower others to run your life.* Instead, empower yourself to get what you want. Staying with the man who begrudges love day after day ensures a diet of "mouthfuls of humiliation." Remaining at a job that limits your potential saps energy and stifles goal setting. The world is full of possibilities and a wealth of rewards for your efforts. Be grateful for the gift of *life*, if you will, and take it from there!

## TRAP #3: SHE DIDN'T GET IT, HOW COULD I?

If you live by making comparisons with what others have accomplished, you won't have time to pay attention to the marvels *you* can work with what you've got. Brooding over your rival's/mentor's/idol's newest failure will surely result in your own lack of success, and soon enough you'll be tripping over yet another hurdle.

How do you fall into this trap? It begins with an inflated vision that *others* have more, are better connected, are smarter, are as meltingly perfect as a pot of honey is to a warm croissant, know the tricks to competing for a prize, have a sturdier psyche, are born graced and lucky. Since you consider these people superior, you stay on guard, mindful of their behavior. Their triumphs you anticipate; their failures shock you. This kind of thinking is murderously effective. "With all her background, Mary can't find a job," you say to yourself. "What kind of fool would I be to give the same dream a chance for myself?"

To climb out of this trap, you'll need to do a little sleuthing. Start by knowing what goals your "ideal" person *didn't* achieve. Perhaps Mary wasn't taken on for a plum job—the very kind of position you'd love to get. Ask yourself these questions: Did she present herself to the prospective employer far too flamboyantly, too eagerly, too aggressively? Could she have revealed a major flaw that would be incompatible with functioning on the job? Was she overqualified or underqualified? Is she really someone who follows through or just makes a lot of noise about having authority and organizational skills? Could she be capable of diabolical plotting to get what she wants—and been tripped up this time?

How on earth does *her* inability to fulfill a goal really reflect on your future happiness? Root around and find the truth.

A little shrewdness will be invaluable to you here. You want to figure out who this ideal person is and why you feel ill-equipped to compete with her, if that's the case. By perpetuating the image of the supposedly superior person, you may be creating *imaginary* competition. This will prevent you from developing on your own.

By now you must have noticed that there are a lot of volunteers who are living your life for you. Some take the direct approach: "I'll tell you when you need a new winter coat." "You're too fat for tap-dancing lessons." "You don't need psychotherapy, you just need to relax." These helpful types are endlessly absorbed with controlling your actions and reactions. They're often happy to report how someone "better" didn't get what you wanted.

Other volunteers are first-rate manipulators. They want to charm you into feeling self-doubt or deliver a backhanded compliment, then control you. "When are you going to get a decent salary to go with that fancy title?" "You're so thrifty: I bet you saved all your size

eighteens for when you gain back that sixty pounds."
"Oh, I'm sorry! I thought you were the salesgirl, not
someone who shopped here."

All of us in this trap react to the idea that we are
inadequate to the task. We even listen attentively when
we're told just that. Those who have an investment in
our staying the same are quick to reinforce our doubts
—this is simply a fact of life. That's why the smart
cookie lengthens her stride, sets her standards, *accurately* measures herself and others by them—and builds
her confidence to go for the goal no matter what
someone else's experience has been.

## TRAP #4: I'M TOO OLD, IT'S TOO LATE, AND I PROBABLY COULDN'T DO IT ANYWAY

Let me tell you about the seventy-three-year-old
New England man who runs the twenty-six-mile Boston
marathon in an enviable time of under three hours. Or
of the sixty-eight-year-old Virginia woman who was
determined to have a master potter teach her his
craft—a master who was located in the hills of Korea.
That she was obliged to leave her comfortable home
and move into primitive quarters to be near him for one
year was never the issue. What mattered was making
pottery.

Age and circumstance, in most cases, have little to do
with fulfilling a dream. Think about it. A woman in her
thirties, forties, fifties and sixties—and why not older?
—can still have the energy and enthusiasm to open a
business, write a novel, design a clothing collection, go
back to school for any degree, even start medical
school.

Of course there are certain physical truths about
basic life functions, and sometimes it *will* be too late. If

you are past menopause, no amount of planning or wishing can get you pregnant with the child you always wanted. It is not too late, though, to adopt a child. So, do you want the child and the joy it will bring or do you prefer the feeling of deprivation that comes with being deep within this trap?

There will be other truths, not necessarily biological, that will help you find an effective way to get what you want—or an equally satisfying substitute. To do so, examine the rules and attitudes you follow—rules and attitudes that may be outdated, arbitrary and not in your best interest at all.

This trap is fascinating in its operation. It can start influencing you in your early twenties and rule you until your last breath: "I'm twenty-three, with two small kids. I have no time for myself." "I'm thirty-three and have no energy left after helping my husband with his business." "I'm forty-three and too old to learn a profession." "I'm fifty-three and want a divorce, but I'm too scared of the consequences." "I'm sixty-three, bored and lonely." And on and on.

The major function of this trap is to block or prevent change by establishing an unbeatable defense (what can I do about my age?) against moving forward. It has an uncanny ability to tell you what you *should* do while limiting what you *can* do. For some of you, the trap clearly creates a conflict. You recognize that it wants you to give up on your life, but something nagging inside you says, dream on. You can dream on once you recognize that it's not too late to immerse yourself in the extraordinary process of living, the ongoing beauty of life.

A friend recently toasted me on my birthday and commented wryly, "May you get all your wishes but one." Surprised, I asked him why. "So you always have something to strive for," he replied. Sounds smart to me.

## TRAP #5: I NEED OTHERS TO DO IT FOR ME

Not long ago, a divorced friend told me she had an idea that could possibly change the shopping habits of a large community—improve sales, in fact—by setting up uniquely structured child-care centers in malls. Tina combined her everyday experiences of being a mother (limited in shopping time because of her small children) with being a good researcher and came up with a plan that allowed mothers more shopping time. It sounded good.

Tina encountered a number of obstacles as she sought financial backing, enough starting money to open one of these centers. We met for lunch; I listened. Tina's arguments were persuasive. She produced charts and figures; the centers would work but what she needed was a break—contact with a man I knew who built shopping malls. If he'd invest in a center, she could make it work.

In her efforts to encourage my support, she noted in a skillful and charming way that sometimes all it takes for success is the right contact at the right time. I concurred, and I was willing to help.

I made the call to meet the gentleman in question; he heard me out. Though he was not swept away by the estimated profits he'd take in from such centers, the project appealed to him on a personal, humanitarian level. What could be more perfect for Tina—an investor with a philanthropic streak!

What was next? Tina had to call him, set up meetings and present her charts, figures, impressions, alternative plans and get his signature on a check. It was here that I backed out—child-care centers and their operation were *Tina's* specialty. Only she never called and of course the investor never pursued her.

Tina dropped the project, pleading lack of time because of a newly formed relationship with a man, but encouraged me to continue. By backing off, she restored her sense of control over the trap she's in. She hoped others would leave her current lifestyle intact and not threaten the relationship she was immersed in. Meanwhile, she's passed up an important chance by hoping that others would make her dream come true for her.

This trap has a close relative: the idea that *success* happens only to others. Those who believe others have "all the luck" find ways to confirm their beliefs. Any personal attainment of good fortune or overnight success, great or small, is played down and diminished by the theory that "magic" only touches others.

"All the luck" often means that others do not make an effort but have good fortune bestowed upon them. In some cases on this earth it is blatantly so. Monarchs, movie stars and "movers and shakers" get what they want an enviably high percentage of the time.

The rest of us must plan judiciously, learn how to use contacts and skills and try to meet our destiny with some sense of humor. Hard work and luck, though, can go together—*the harder you work the luckier you get.* When you act—that is, do what you care about—you stir up life, meet people, increase opportunities, even collide joyfully with those fateful "lucky" moments.

To bring the concept down to a simple analogy: It's the difference between giving a man a fish or teaching him how to fish. Give him the fish and he'll have to wait for the next one. "If he's lucky," you'll come around with the day's catch when he's hungry. But what of the man with the skill to ensure his own survival, who can fish in any waters? I think you know the answer.

## TRAP #6: IT'S THEIR GAME, BUT I HAVE TO PLAY IT WITH MY RULES

A patient tells me that she's struggling to understand the complicated politics of the unit she works in at a large hospital. Her struggle, she says, has altered her disposition, her sleeping habits, her style of coping, to a noticeable level. She still loves her job, though it's become more a matter of mastering stress and artful manipulation of co-workers and higher-ups than doing the work she excels at. Unraveling the politics of an organization is a common pastime out there in the world of business, but to Marianne, the machinations at the hospital unit seem especially dire.

With this amount of information about Marianne, you might suppose that she's fearful of being fired or quitting a good thing. Not quite.

The very higher-ups whom Marianne broods over are thrilled with her; they have offered her a major promotion. She was flattered, having had her eye on this job for a long time and sorely wanting it. Now it could be hers. Or not hers. She turned it down!

The surface reasons Marianne gave for the turndown were: too much bookkeeping (she was a ninny with figures) and too many committee meetings (her coping mechanism was marginal at best; how did they expect her to be an ambassador of goodwill?).

But the real reason is characteristic of women caught in this trap: Given the opportunity to reach a goal, they respond by backing down because the situation does not match their fixed and rather prejudiced view of how the game should be played.

The hospital, in Marianne's case, did not see fit to adapt itself to her rules. Marianne has a different game in mind. In her fantasy hospital unit there is always fair play, she can shrug off those irritating little things that pop up each day, and those who can deal with numbers work on balancing the budget and don't bother her. In this dream unit, Marianne's blood pressure is lower than everyone else's.

The fantasy unit doesn't exist, but the promotion does. Unless Marianne starts up her own hospital, establishes her own modus operandi and hires a staff who must comply or leave, she will have to learn how to play the game according to real-life rules. No matter what hospital she works in, there will be politics, stress, personal idiosyncrasies, and promotions for the taking, but Marianne refuses to accept that.

Her story has an interesting conclusion. The woman hired for the job, Marianne's rival, lasted about six months, then transferred out. Marianne was again offered the job.

This time she stepped into the promotion. In understanding the difference between acceptance and denial, she had developed a far more commendable attitude and was showing some responsibility for herself: she wanted the job and now she was willing to take what came with it. The predominant motivation was to get her life off hold. Marianne understood, finally, that her future could only duplicate her past unless she was willing to take the risk. Proudly, she did.

## TRAP #7: IT'S NOT THE RIGHT TIME

After a flurry of unsuccessful attempts over the past few years to leave her husband, Ted, Audrey still lives with him, continuing her pattern of alternately seething in anger or going through the motions of accommodation. Ted is usually either psychologically or financially in trouble, depending on whether he's working or not, or whether he's punishing and begrudging toward Audrey to keep her, he assumes, "in line."

Though Ted's behavior is generally upsetting most of the time, he can be charming, boyish, tender and sexually arousing to Audrey—giving just enough to prevent her from seriously demanding that he leave. Audrey is proud of her forgiving response—"nobody's perfect"—until Ted persists in his special kind of torture. He is good at disappearing for eight-hour clips, offering no explanations. So, couple his pattern of only sporadically contributing to the household finances with his psychologically cruel behavior, and Audrey crumbles—she wants him out.

How does she tell him?

Audrey sits him down and tells him she understands his problems—he's having rough times in business, his mother was just hospitalized, he's very sensitive and needs a drink to reduce tension—but when is he going to change? When will he shape up?

Ted is fond of these impassioned speeches. They actually move him, watching Audrey's vast reservoir of "understanding" defy all laws of nature: no matter how much she uses, the pool remains undrained. Ted shapes up for a while, deluding Audrey into thinking they have harmonious goals. Then something unpleasant happens in his life and he's back to being Ted. And Audrey again wonders what it would feel like to be single again at thirty-eight. She wants him to leave.

I repeat my question: How does she ask him to leave?

She doesn't—not quite. Because *it's never the right time.* Here's why, according to Audrey's reasoning.

Ted's business suffers seasonal setbacks, so it's not a good time *off*-season to ask him for a divorce. He's already hurt. *On*-season, he's cheerful a good deal and openhanded with money, so it's the time to encourage him, not request that he turn in his house key. Ted suffers from depression (he likes to sleep away most of the weekends), allergies or hangovers. It's not the right time when he's feeling sick.

To sum up: When Ted's vulnerable, Audrey doesn't want to add to his emotional burdens. And when Ted shapes up, he meets Audrey's requirements for a good husband and therefore she won't show him the door. Neither circumstance is flattering to Audrey's self-esteem. Ted has what he wants: a hold on Audrey strong enough to satisfy him. And Audrey, remarkably susceptible to Ted's manipulations, is stuck on hold.

What's in this marriage for Ted? He gets what he wants—a chance to live to the peak of his immaturity. He's chosen his wife well, too. She's an *enabler:* someone who scolds him, threatens him, but essentially encourages—not discourages—his childish behavior patterns. Ted can provoke guilt in Audrey when she demands that he participate more fully in the marriage. Why? Because he is, remember, always down on his luck, or suffering along with a parent, or wheezing from some unnamed virus or whatever has struck him a blow "from behind." *It's never the right time.*

Audrey would like to find the right time. As she envisions it, Ted would commit some unpardonable act that would goad her over the edge. Falling, she'd call out, "Pack your things and be out in one hour!" It is crisis alone, Audrey confesses to me, that could get her to actually utter the words.

This trap ensnares so many women who mistake a husband's "vulnerability" for what it really is—the weapons of the weak. And they are potent weapons, especially when aimed in your direction.

There's a guiding principle that can help women to take the first step out of this trap: Realize that the right time is when it's *the right time for you*, not for him. The right time has to do with a willingness to let go of what's holding you back. The right time is when you know, deep down, that it's time to get your life off hold.

## TRAP #8: I WANT SOMETHING BUT I DON'T KNOW WHAT IT IS

Betty confides to me that her life is like living in a "falling-rock zone" where she's constantly pelted by reminders of neglected projects, all-consuming jealousies, excruciating feelings of guilt at her inactivity, disproportionate values put on chores, fantasies of the happiness that has been denied her. While this avalanche gathers momentum, Betty stands willingly by, hoping her knees won't buckle under the daily pileup. *But someday the moment will come when she can decide what to do with her life*. Then, finally, she'll be able to step aside from the bombardment and be free to be herself.

This is Betty's trap: She cannot define what she wants. Instead, she buries all possibilities in a muddle of confusion, under an avalanche of feelings, muffed opportunities and overlooked choices. Not unlike Mr. Micawber in *David Copperfield*, Betty lives without direction, waiting around, as Mrs. Micawber pointed out about her husband, "in case anything turns up, which was his favorite expression."

Betty wants something, but what? Why doesn't she know what it is? Too many choices out there? Not enough choices? "Ten years ago," Betty explained, "I just wanted to be happy, but something was always missing. I never knew what. Now I feel I'm supposed to grow as a person and don't know how."

Probably you've figured out that Betty's unrealized ambitions—being happy or being her most productive self—will remain unrealized until she's willing to *define her goals*. As is the case with many such women, Betty has the misguided notion that the act of describing a goal, feeling, attitude or action makes it less valuable, less powerful, or less interesting. Or, that by defining it at all, she will be obliged to proceed with carrying it out at any cost.

If she looked a little closer, she could see that clarification bestows power. By clinging stubbornly to a vague idea of "something," Betty can never accomplish anything or find her happiness.

Making life choices is an intensely individual matter. No one can ever be more ambitious for you than you are for yourself. Betty and other women who share the compelling attraction of this particular trap may well be ambitious, but they never have to face what they can't define.

The solution for climbing out of this trap? Come up with a clearly defined plan for what you want and prepare an active reason for why you should have it! Devise a dream, a mission, a five-year plan—make it simple or intricately plotted. To do this, picture what would please you most. Begin the image by saying to yourself, "I would enjoy . . ." and fill in the blanks. What do you see yourself doing? Paint in the details as richly as you can, and encourage emotionally vivid descriptions. Let it excite you. List the steps that you might take to begin getting what you want. Be creative.

You can even define what you want by listing what *dis*pleases you most ("I don't want to be poor anymore"; "I can't bear another moment with Harry"), which is approaching goals, to be blunt, from the back door. But open this door if it will lead you to another entrance—a positive plan of action. Remember this in any case: Decisions can be changed. Decisions can be tailored to fit. One mistaken decision is not an omen signifying a lifetime of disappointments.

Marlo Thomas said something wonderful in an interview with me. Speaking of her relationship with husband Phil Donahue, Marlo revealed how she defined herself and her career goals to him before they married. Her statement made perfect sense. "I am as ambitious as you," she told him. "I want for myself what you want for yourself. I want you to think of me as you think of yourself and you'll know who I am."

Clearly, here is a woman who won't be caught in the "I-don't-know-what-I-want" trap—a smart cookie!

# Taking the First Steps to Getting Your Life Off Hold

"People often commit themselves to the idea of change, but not to the *effort* of change," says Dr. William Knaus in his interesting book *How to Conquer Your Frustrations*. "As a result, they fail to properly assess their situation, to carefully identify achievable goals, to formulate plans, to organize for action, and to put the plans into action."

The eight traps, I've found, are the most immediate problems women face—traps that can stifle or excuse away the effort to get your life off hold. Can you add to these traps? Do you worry about pleasing others first, for example, rather than improving a bad situation you are in? Does your decision about whether or not to take your life off hold reflect a fear of doing things alone? By looking at what happens to you when you feel that impulse to stop—by being aware that you have just fallen into a trap—you can start assessing your situation and get your life off hold.

Jane, whose case I cited earlier, turned down an opportunity for medical school. Lost opportunities and bottled-up feelings of deprivation are two consequences of the fear-of-success/fear-of-failure trap. The knowledge that she could take responsibility for her life did not stand up under her scrutiny. She panicked. Jane did not want to take responsibility for her problems, at least not yet. Faulty rationales kept her on hold.

Though Jane muffed her chances, at least she could identify her goal exactly—medical school. Many women worry that they have no goal, that they have no skills for identifying choices. Others feel so enfolded by the traps that keep them on hold that they are confused by the weightiness of making life choices. Still others don't know what questions to ask to solve problems in relationships or work.

Consider all the predicaments involved in keeping your life on hold, and now think of feeling good as you empty those traps and start to rebuild your future. To do that, you have to learn more about yourself and *underline* how you deal with specific issues. How do you, or don't you, put plans into action? Take this quiz. It's designed to help you analyze the course of your life and assist you in clarifying why you get stuck on hold. Answers will reveal your feelings and attitudes about taking action to create a true change. The final section will direct you in making some choices that can transform your life.

First, let's see how you feel about some troublesome

emotional issues that could be influencing your life and keeping you on hold. Your feelings and how you express them are unique to you. Be honest with yourself.

### 1. *Feelings and Interactions*

* Do you tend to hide from yourself?
* Do you find that facing a crisis brings out negative feelings?
* Do you pretend to like things that displease you to gain the approval of others?
* Do you tend to blame yourself and get depressed because things aren't the way you want them to be?
* If the answer is yes to the previous question, are you unable to take steps to improve the circumstances, so you feel helpless?
* Do you feel afraid right before you take on a task?
* Do people demonstrate a lack of respect for you?
* Can others easily make you feel guilty?
* When others make you feel guilty, do you respond to them with anger?
* Do you find yourself confiding in people who predictably don't offer you comfort, but seem pleased you're not getting what you want?
* Do you blame others for what's wrong in your life?
* Do you feel basically dissatisfied with your life—that it's generally out of control?
* Do you feel uncomfortable when you try to tell people about yourself?
* Do you tend to dramatize events so that you

always appear to be put upon, taken advantage of, or victimized by others?

• Do you have trouble letting others know what you want from them in a direct and honest fashion?

• Would you say that you cannot assert yourself if you feel offended, neglected or passed over for something you want?

• Do you feel uneasy or fearful of the consequences after you've asserted yourself?

Answering yes to most of the questions indicates that you're probably running your life from a position of vulnerability. You feel bruised by life, a little confused about the authenticity of your feelings for others, and, sometimes, overwhelmed by waves of self-doubt. It's this self-doubt that keeps you on hold.

It's time for a reappraisal of your situation. If you are constantly under another's thumb, or are treated in ways that do not please you, or maintain the stance of "the blamer"—that is, events and people are responsible for your life—you may not even know how to start changing. In that case, read on. Let's see how you approach the everyday necessity of making choices.

## 2. *Making Choices*

• Do you feel you have few choices open to you and that you are incapable of acting on them?

• Do you become angry when questioned about some of the choices you've made?

• Do you want the permission of others before acting on the choices you've made?

• Do you expect to be perfect in the execution of those choices?

• Do you deny you really have any choices, feel trapped in the position you find yourself in now?

• Are you unhappy about not being able to make a choice at all?

• Do you try to impose choices on others and control their behavior?

• If you go ahead and make choices for others without consulting them, are you angry or insulted when they complain?

• Do you tend to conceal situations in which there are choices to be made?

• Do you feel you live in a world where others impose on you their idea of which choices you can or can't make?

• Are you easily talked into choices that please you less and others more?

• Do you have trouble seeing yourself living out a choice you want to make?

• Do you back out of competition because you think your choice is actually too much for you, beyond your reach?

• Do you ever wish you could make a choice and go for it just to see if you could get it?

What happened when you answered these questions? Were you uneasy about the process of making choices or were you able to answer the questions decisively? Most of us go through feelings of doubt about the choices we make. Why?

Making choices means you may not get an immediate reward, but does imply that you are aiming for the pleasure of long-term benefits. How do you make choices to realize those rewards and benefits? If you let others make them for you, you have already chosen to surrender control of your life. You are too vulnerable to suggestion, following a course others design for you. If you make decisions for others so that you *do not* have to act, creating situations in which others succeed *for* you, you have chosen to keep your life on hold.

You may be intuitively aware that certain choices will change your life, but they seem threatening. You wonder who you are, who you'll be, if you make those choices. So let's take a closer look at your qualities.

### 3. *Describe Yourself*

| | |
|---|---|
| Loving | Fair |
| Warm | Foolish |
| Emotionally distant | Childish |
| Adventurous | Complaining |
| Timid | Sarcastic |
| Shy | Feel powerful |
| Enthusiastic | Feel powerless |
| High energy | Lack confidence |
| Lack energy | Feel cheated |
| Quick-tempered | Attractive |
| Frequently angry | Unattractive |
| Easy disposition | Sexy |
| Good-humored | Not sexy |
| Cheerful | Perfectionist |
| Smart | Spendthrift |
| Not smart | Compulsive eater |
| Decisive | |

Which qualities have you checked off? Would you like to meet the person you've described, feeling she's someone who reaches out to others? Select the qualities that you want to develop and the ones you want to minimize. Write these down and describe situations in which they cause you satisfaction or displeasure.

Some of these qualities may generate denial: "No, I couldn't be quick-tempered. Everyone provokes me, is all!" Or hesitation: "I'm not sure if I complain all the time or not." In that case, enlist a friend and have her tell you when she thinks those qualities manifest themselves. The first step to unlearning a type of behavior is to be aware of it in action.

Since you are a complex individual, you have certain essential needs. Let's identify them next.

If you feel a need listed below is not very important, assign it #1; if the need is moderately important, rank it #2; and if the need is very important, give it #3. This system can help you see what's required for your basic survival.

4. *Your Needs*

to feel productive
for privacy
to belong
for self-confidence
for challenge
for independence
for perfection
for power
to be loving
to be conscientious
to be controlled

for social contact
to feel safe
to learn
to be right
to trust in yourself
for competence
to show emotion
to avoid trouble
to give in
to acquire possessions
to control others

What you want to strive for here is a *balance*. One need in itself should not stand alone or neurotically reduce the importance of another. When a need becomes obsessive, perceptions are distorted. It can take you over, and you will let nothing get in the way of satisfying it. Once you know which needs are important to basic survival, you can say yes to them. For example, I need privacy, but I also understand that sometimes there will be disruptions. When they happen, I've learned to cope with the disruptions and not let them rattle my composure.

This list of needs may help you with another point—how to make decisions based on the degree of importance of your needs. Here's what I mean. You are a woman who has assigned #3 (very important) to the "need to belong." Your marriage is foundering, and, while you contemplate divorce, you feel marriage is a refuge, better than being out in the cold. In this case, you should decide to work on reducing the importance of the need before you make a move. Examine how "belonging" in a bad marriage constitutes a refuge for you. Can you slowly begin to shift the focus from belonging in a bad marriage to belonging to yourself, and then to others? (We'll talk more about that in the next chapter.)

Perhaps what's keeping you on hold are the expectations you have for yourself. See which ones affect you.

## 5. *Clarify Your Expectations*

• For this exercise, pick out one person who matters in your life—a person whose approval you need. Make two columns—one that will list what you expect of yourself and one that will list what you think the other person expects of you concerning the same matter.

I've supplied nine common expectations for you to start with. Think about which others influence the form of your life.

Expectations have everything to do with how we see ourselves. They can be limited or expansive, unrealistic or realistic, disruptive or unifying, short range or long range. The same rules of self-understanding apply to expectations as to needs. If we expect too much (or become too needy) we encourage limitation, not expansiveness, and we bend to get approval rather than venturing out.

| *Yourself* | *Him/Herself* |
| --- | --- |
| I expect to marry and be committed to making the marriage work. | |
| I expect not to marry and get along well enough. | |
| I expect not to marry and eventually regret it. | |
| I expect my mother/father to be there always to bail me out of difficulties. | |
| I expect my husband to feel warm and loving toward me all the time. | |
| I expect my husband to give me what I want to make me happy. | |
| I expect to not have children but focus on a career. | |
| I expect to have a career and inte- | |

grate it with my roles as wife and
mother.

I expect my career to cause a
strain on my family.

Our expectations can get us into trouble and create
guilt when we take on more than we can achieve.
Suppose you expect to have a career and children. This
clashes with your husband's point of view on the
matter—he wants you home. What to do? Create a
balance sheet. What are the pluses you can cite to him?
If you work, you can afford to hire cleaning help and
babysitters; you can contribute to a downpayment on a
new car, a trip abroad, his mother's coming surgery
bill. In what way can you show him that *his* expectations can be expanded to include your career since they
benefit him, too? Now tally up the down side of the
balance sheet, including your guilts: Your husband is
angry about the absence (or lateness) of hot meals at
dinnertime since you started working (that makes you
feel bad); your mother calls every other day to remind
you what a bad mother you are (you feel negligent and
angry). And so on.

Start balancing your life's expectations. Understand
that you cannot change the way everyone feels, thinks
and responds to you. You cannot expect to change
everyone around you so that things will go your way.
You cannot expect of others what you are unwilling to
do for or give yourself. You cannot expect "if" to solve
your problems: "If" you say the right thing your
husband will be a kinder man; "if" you stay home, your
daughter will be a paragon of girlhood and your mother
will respect and adore you. Unfortunately, this is an

unreasonable level of expectation. It's never going to happen.

For life to be taken off hold, for it to be a vivid adventure—and why shouldn't it be!—start now to free yourself from dissatisfactions, the old grievances and expectations, the needs that make up your private experience. Consolation is not enough—I know you're all struggling to rise from what you were (or are) to what you could be. I've felt similar frustrations myself.

But how good it will feel to say to someone you care for, "This is the path I've decided to take. I want you *in* my life, but understand that you can never *be* my life, live my life, or keep my life on hold."

# 2

---

# Wearing the Cloak of Inferiority

Clare was raised by a mother who begrudged her affection, positive attention, emotional support. Even when she was very young, Clare could not figure out what she'd done wrong to earn such constant reproaches. She tried so hard to please her mother, but somehow she never got the knack. If she was asked to perform some household task, Clare did so agreeably and eagerly. Then, a moment later, her mother would tell Clare in condescending tones to forget it—*she* would do it and do it better and more efficiently instead. Clare was never, in her mother's eyes, competent, bright, or pretty enough. Clare could never make the right decision or be happy with what she was given. If her mother bought her two blouses and Clare tried one on for fit, her mother would sneer, "I see the other wasn't good enough for you."

Rather than be a defiant daughter, Clare put all her efforts into pleasing her mother. This often proved impossible. The woman never quite allowed Clare the satisfaction of knowing she could be pleased. As she grew older, Clare more and more believed her mother's opinions of her—that she was a basically worthless human being who occupied far too much space. "I felt as if I'd been wrapped in a cloak of inferiority," she said, "sitting alone, going nowhere."

When she was twenty-one, she was still trying to gain her mother's love. She attempted to please her mother now by finding a "catch" of a man, to prove to her mother that she was worth something by being loved by "someone." The man she elected to marry was a doctor, a handsome, charming man to whom the words marital fidelity were unknown. For ten years of their marriage, he dated other women, apologetic to Clare, but not caring enough to stop his philandering. Clare divorced him. With her two small children, she moved back to her parents' home, where her mother resumed her tirades. Clare, she said, wasn't clever enough to hold a man—hadn't she always told her that?

A few years later, Clare met another man—cut from the same cloth as her first husband. He, too, cheated on Clare and she finally asked for a divorce after five years. Maybe her mother was right all along, she thought. Maybe she wasn't enough of a woman to keep an interesting man interested.

This time she didn't return to her parents' home, but stayed in the apartment where she'd been living. She learned hairdressing and worked, successfully, at a shop for five years, supporting her children, but hesitant about marrying again. Her mother, all this while, reminded her that if she were a better person, there'd be a man to support her and the children and she wouldn't have to stoop to working in a blue-collar trade.

Clare was lonely, though, and aware of her mistakes in choosing the dashing womanizers. Next time, she swore to herself, she'd find a nice, stable guy who would never leave her. At forty-four she did just that. Her third husband is a kindhearted man, but dull, slight, not particularly attractive to her; a man who makes an adequate enough living. He adores Clare; he's thrilled, in fact, that a woman as pretty and competent as Clare has chosen *him*. He is, in a way, who she was in her first two marriages—the one who feels gifted by the presence of a "superior" being who makes him feel less inferior.

Clare's been married to her third husband for fifteen years, but she's still holding on to a dream—the dream of marrying a dynamic, successful, attractive man who will adore her. It's also her wish to garner the strength to get out of this marriage before it's too late and she's too old to really enjoy life. Her mother, still going strong, assures Clare that it will never happen.

A sad story, this one—the kind that has many variations among women who go from overpowering parents to denying spouses. Neither parents nor spouses can be pleased—that much is evident. Neither want their victims to be strong—and they make sure it's weakness, compliancy, that they get.

A mother like Clare's has an extraordinary effect on how her daughter lives and the choices she makes. How can her influence be ignored? Clare's history records negative messages about her abilities to perform, her looks, her lovableness in general—and all had been found wanting by her mother. In trying to prove her lovableness, she selected men her mother would deem superior. Known then by the company she was keeping, Clare would finally be seen by Mother as being worthy of caring and attention. Clare's first marriage pleased her mother only on selfish terms—she could tell others that her son-in-law was a doctor. Clare got little credit for the matches, and little sympathy came her way for her divorces and the reasons behind them. To her mother, Clare was at fault—a disgrace in fact.

This weighty cloak of inferiority around Clare's shoulders is a garment common among women who were raised as Clare was. If we've worn one, we wonder why and how it got there in the first place. One explanation goes this way: When we were very young, we needed parental protection, care, love and guidance. We learned what in the world was safe for us, what signaled danger. The limits of our universe were described to us and we were to stay within those limits. This was a time when we learned, too, if we were lovable or not and how to get what we needed from the world. Some parents, then, took the nurturing of children to mean domination and total control. They used their power as adults and twisted it unmercifully to break down a child's will, undermine her, humiliate her. Children were controlled by mothers (or fathers) who thought that a show of affection, enthusiasm for a child's abilities or dreams, or tenderness of any sort loosened the grip they had on the young lives they were molding. They wanted the child to feel inferior.

Now sixty years old, Clare is still trying to please an octogenarian mother who will not approve of her. This mother may rightly believe that denigration kept her daughter tied to her, but at what cost to both of them? Here's Clare now: She may still be seeking the ideal man, but she *has* made progress. Though her mother doesn't like it that she works in a beauty salon (and her husband does like it), Clare is finally happy with her work. She has learned a skill and does well at it. She can take care of herself; and her children, now grown, are able to do the same. This counts for her—but that gnawing sense of inferiority still works on her. And her mother, by berating her daughter over a lifetime, has missed the point of intimate relationships, which are not based on tyranny, but compassion.

Clare's mother, in her own hard-as-nails style, is not a woman at peace with herself or terribly sure of her lovableness or competence. She too is an example of a woman with deep-seated feelings of inferiority. As Clare is compliant, openly showing her vulnerability and need for approval, so is her mother dictatorial, afraid of letting others see that she can be hurt, and demanding that others cater to her. Her harshness is intended to create the illusion of superiority and the implication of everyone else's inferiority. What makes this tough cookie tick may appear baffling to those of us more attuned to Clare's manner of coping, but it's not. Basically, the tough cookie functions like this:

She is a woman who wants your hackles to rise. She'll create an environment where malevolence simmers and she's in control. She'll wield hostility to get her way, but it leaves her feeling empty. She's not a good winner; she needs to abuse the loser. If there is an unnamed fear in her soul, it's of being found out—that her conflicts are plentiful, that she's sadly low in self-esteem, that she experiences panicky waves of helplessness, that she may be dressed for success or spend the day in a housecoat, but underneath she wears a cloak of inferiority.

Consider Brenda's story. Married, with two children, Brenda took an executive position in the sales division of a small, upcoming company. Immediately establishing herself as a force to be reckoned with, she was benevolent and malevolent by turns, depending on what she wanted at the moment.

Brenda discovered she could easily dominate the women at the office, except for Caroline, a woman about ten years older who greeted Brenda's chronic belligerence and cynicism with indifference and her angry outbursts with rational discussion. This response bothered Brenda—who was Caroline to treat her democratically, not deferentially? Brenda would not spare her when the time came.

The time came. Brenda's home life was in turmoil. There were complaints about the babysitters from her kids; late-in-the-day laments from her husband, who was in a difficult position at his law firm. In a moment of weakness, Brenda talked about the babysitter problem; Caroline suggested that she hire an older woman, perhaps a retiree, who'd be reliable, experienced, even devoted, rather than the teenage girls, who were frequently disappointing. Brenda found this suggestion profoundly annoying. Beyond that, it was an assault on her judgment in hiring young girls who, she insisted, were easier to mold in her image.

Caroline's position demanded a lot of public speaking, conferences, presentations; Brenda's job kept her in the office. Brenda wanted Caroline's job, or, at the very least, Caroline out of a job. She took to making disparaging comments about Caroline, tried to humiliate her and made her the butt of jokes. ("Caroline thinks she's going over good, but she's making a jerk of herself. So what else is new?" "She wants everyone to love her, but who on earth *could?*" "It does my heart good to see her looking like hell.") Brenda's resentment and jealousy escalated. Her cracks were repeated to Caroline by an ally who thought she should know about Brenda's backstabbing.

Caroline did not confront Brenda in private, but called for a meeting with her and the president of the company, right before Caroline was to renew her contract with the firm. The president was filled in on Brenda's year-long onslaught on Caroline's character and work efforts. Caroline accused Brenda of being unable to accept a compliment or suggestion, of insulting and viciously attacking her behind her back, and of being the worst kind of role model for other young women in the company. Caroline explained that she did not want to leave her job, but neither did she deserve to suffer such indignities. She would be forced to step around Brenda, to the company's detriment, so they'd have as little to do with each other as possible.

To Caroline's surprise, Brenda crumbled. She began crying, then denied she'd said anything to hurt Caroline. Caroline and the president knew she was guilty of at least half of what had been attributed to her—and that was bad enough. Confronted by this delicate situation, she admitted that Caroline was right. She *had* been a bully, a backstabber, a destroyer of team spirit.

Bitterness, belligerence and bickering can signify toughness, even power, to women like Brenda. That amounts to piling on heavy metal armor over an already weighty cloak of inferiority. On the face of it, Brenda is in an excellent position at the company—she was brought in by the president, who saw her worth. Threatened by Caroline's restraint and self-confidence, Brenda covered over her fears by attacking. Caroline was a target to be picked on, to agitate, to downgrade and eventually depose from any position of authority. Under all the noise, Brenda felt weak, insignificant.

Like many other women, she wore a cloak of inferiority, fitted it tightly to herself and didn't realize she didn't need it at all.

Belief in their inferiority is as entrapping as a straitjacket for some women, and they will be lashed into it for life unless someone helps them untie the straps. The cloak of inferiority traps all their fears within its folds: fears that they're not worth knowing, that they're not smart enough, that they have no skills and can't develop any. The cloak magnifies fears that they're not people in their own right, that they can't do anything by themselves and need to be cared for like children. It makes them believe they're not capable of earning money and living on their own; that they're not lovable or pretty enough to attract a man; that it's easier to overeat and gain weight than care for their bodies.

Feeling inferior does not feel good. Among the symptoms are confusion, flash anger, overeating and possibly alcoholism, combativeness and a preoccupation with the past. There may also be a disproportionate fear of the unknown, in which it's as if the unlived future is a lurking nightmare—one false step and you'll tumble into the void, shattered.

A number of women I know come to mind as examples of how these symptoms operate.

Tara, I'd say, almost wills herself into trouble on a fairly regular basis. On the job, she is known to be impulsive, unfocused, and difficult to direct. Rather than asking for guidance when she doesn't know how to solve a problem or how to proceed, she invariably makes the wrong decision. Tara will not ask direct questions, but talks around them, hoping to get the information she needs that way. On the surface, it appears that she takes criticism well—tell her what she's done wrong and she'll nod "yes"—but she's not listening or taking it in; she doesn't want to understand what you're actually saying. Instead, she plunges head-long into her work, often creating more confusion, and sometimes in spite of herself getting it right. To Tara, misguided action is better than admitting she doesn't know what to do. She fears that by asking direct questions, she will not only be demonstrating a lack of knowledge but exposing her inferiority. Others, to her, know more, have more, *are* more.

Dana, on the other hand, cannot take criticism, no matter how insignificant, without putting up a fight. She is driven by a need to be perfect. Point out her mistakes and she becomes breathless, angry. Rather than make the simple correction and go on to something else, she demands to know why her critic did not see what she did *right*. She is furious for not being complimented, and tormented by being corrected. Dana cannot step back to observe the truth of the criticism. Feeling inferior inside, she takes it personally—as if you were saying *she* was the mistake. In her anger, she will continue to defend her error throughout the day—she got the wrong information; others didn't speak clearly so of course she misinterpreted what they said; the typewriter wasn't working. Flash anger and flash fights are her defenses, her way of letting others know she can't be belittled by criticism, while trying to affirm that she's perfect, incapable of making a false move.

Georgette feels a lack of substance to her life—something's missing. It could be love, accomplishment, a direction, a sense of balance between relationships and work, self-concern—or all of them. Georgette, as she tells it, sometimes is "empty," and she solves that gnawing feeling with food. For her, it's the quickest and simplest way to become warm and full. Food dulls her pain temporarily; she no longer feels deprived, inferior, because she has been unable to get what she yearns for. If she gains a lot of weight, that compounds the feelings of inferiority—she looks ungainly, undesirable. Then the vicious cycle takes over. To assuage the anxiety about being overweight, she eats to comfort herself. The result: She's exactly where she started when she took that first bite to dull her pain.

Wendy tends to fret over the past, making it a perpetual model for the present and future. To Wendy, her shortcomings and failures are far more meaningful than her abilities and strengths. She reminds herself through flashbacks that she's never done this or that right before, so she has no expectancy of doing it right or better now or ever. She's got the record to prove it. Wendy reacts as though everything in the present and potential future has already happened in the past. By this logic, she is doomed. The future, a different and better future, frightens her. What if she can't cope with having what she wants; what if it's snatched from her? So she lives in the past, reinforcing her feelings of inferiority. Wendy is unable to cut off the past and say "so what!" to those mistakes, turning them around to use them as learning experiences for improving the future.

Though Wendy resides in the past and dreads the future without true cause, some women are justified in fearing the unknown—the woman with small children who wants to leave an abusive husband naturally wonders who will care for them without his assistance. But fear need not hold her back. Rather, caution, planning and a reliable support system can guide her step by step out of the hole she's in.

Women who wear the cloak of inferiority often unconsciously look for other people, including husbands, who will buttress their fears. At bottom, the abused wife mentioned above wants her husband to be a good father and a responsible husband. But she may select a man who thinks first, last, and always of himself.

She may have a husband who has never reconciled himself to marriage, who stays out late, philanders, makes his wife beg for money. A patient in a situation like this once told me: "I knew he wasn't much when I married him, but I never expected it to be *this* bad!" Frank is not a husband to Janine: after seven years of marriage, he still considers himself a single man encumbered by a woman who declares herself his wife while two small beings who look like him call him Daddy. Janine won't leave the marriage, bad as it is, because she believes in her inferiority, her inability to "do any better" than Frank.

When, like Janine, you wear the cloak of inferiority, you tend to walk with your head bowed, never daring to look at two simple axioms up there on the horizon: *Do not expect a man to show you more respect than he shows for himself. Do not expect a man to give you respect when you're content with disrespect.*

Janine suffers from a common dilemma. She wants to shake off the cloak of inferiority, lighten the load on her shoulders, and have Frank treat her with respect. Since she's still wearing the cloak, she tells me with lowered eyes that "Frank knows me too well . . . I can't change."

To shake off the cloak, you must listen very carefully to what you tell yourself about who you are. Are you parroting what your parents, husband, friends, have told you? Do you really *believe* what you're hearing? Or can you change?

While there is no magical leap from feeling inferior to having an idyllic marriage, a great job, enviable children or first prize in the Pillsbury bake-off, there is a formula for feeling good about yourself. By giving yourself positive reminders of the good things you do and the good qualities you have, you can then allow yourself to take *small steps* toward a goal and let those small steps *count*. Do not beat yourself up for mistakes, for lapses of discipline, for small forgetfulnesses. When you meet a goal, no matter how small, that cloak of inferiority is closer to dropping off. And there are ways to help shake it. Let's take a look at some of the things you can do to replace negativity with energizing feelings of worthiness.

# Don't Accept That Others Know You Better Than You Know Yourself

All it takes is the memory of one voice. Think about it. Whom do you hear uttering opinions about your creative, financial or physical limitations, or the boundaries of your personality? Is that reproving "I know better" edge to the voice as trenchant this moment as it was the first time you heard it?

The owner of the earlier, original voice may no longer exist, but another one, an equally powerful substitute, may still be inhibiting your confidence level. Your husband's voice. A friend's. The neighbors'. At this stage, one of the voices that may automatically be joining in to block you from taking action is *your own*.

You may be sabotaging your efforts as effectively as

anyone else without being fully aware that you're doing it. How does this happen?

Those original messages—the judgments and evaluations made by parents and siblings early in life—have become a potent part of you. "You can't," "You never could," "You're not bright/pretty/talented or deserving enough," they repeated to you over and over again. You may have believed them back then, and now they are a part of you. These judgments play like a tape in your consciousness, but now it's *you* repeating those same negative messages, reinforcing others' faulty, manipulative opinions.

That "I know better" implication may not be a way of "protecting" you, as others claim, but a way to keep you as you are. It's subtle sabotage—sometimes on a conscious level, sometimes not. Here's how:

Since she was a child, a patient's mother has intoned again and again, "You're living in the city of lost hope," whenever Marcia expressed a desire to be an artist. "Imagine you making anything of yourself," a father said with ill-concealed contempt to his daughter, Paula, now a close friend of mine. The "knowing" by others starts with parents, then the range can broaden.

Those who have it in their best interest to discourage your ambitions or encourage doubts about your ability to function—parents, spouse, lovers, friends, siblings, teachers, employers—may need you to fulfill their own selfish needs. They may size up your weaknesses and remind you that you need their support. These are the people who "know" you. They want you to believe that a minefield of perils lies in wait for you unless you walk gingerly with your arm linked with theirs while going in their direction. They know exactly where you may trip up. (They "know" you.) And it is no surprise if they revel in your failures. It proves they are right.

If you are like Marcia, you will sporadically take out your paints. Working makes you feel bad about "defying" your mother (who has no understanding of your creative impulses), while *not* working at the easel increases your feelings of distress about betraying your talent. Your mother, you say to yourself, was right— you lack discipline . . . direction . . . inspired genius . . . an independence of mind to live as an artist.

If you think as Paula does, you're ahead of the game. You've learned how to turn the negative voices off, or certainly lower the pitch to a barely audible hum. Paula has caught on to a truth: The measure of her self-esteem is determined by self-knowledge, not the opinions of others. It was a fight for her. It meant summoning the strength to leave her parents' home, move to another town and begin what eventually became a successful career in advertising. She's not yet free of those haunting voices that point out her shortcomings or entreat her to be "the Paula we know," but that's okay. She knows who she is.

# Learn to Take Criticism

Criticism strikes each of us in profoundly different ways. It may merely make us flinch, or perhaps we usually ignore it and continue behaving as we wish. But for some women wrapped in the cloak of inferiority, being criticized is like being attacked by a SWAT team . . . they feel assaulted, defenseless, and their self-esteem is depleted. An offhand comment may bring them to tears; a boss's year-end evaluation of their capabilities and potential may hurt them so much that they are prompted to quit. Such an oversensitive reaction is unfortunate because they can't look objectively at the criticism, evaluate it and learn from it.

In this life, we need to learn how to steer toward a goal, not into a wall. If you maintain an inviolate sensitivity to criticism and insulate yourself from those who can teach you something, you'll get to know each and every crevice of every wall you hit, and your growth will be thwarted.

It's a popular misconception that criticism is always aimed at leveling those who are being criticized, when in fact some of our critics are sincere and really want to help us. To become a smart cookie, you must be shrewd, aware of the difference between those who are pulling for you and those who aren't. (We already identified one such faction that does not want you to thrive—those who "know you better than you know yourself.")

People are fond of saying about tennis or golf technique, "You don't change a winning stroke." But even a winning stroke can be refined—as any champion will tell you. To them, each round presents a challenge to learn the game anew. They view films of their performances, endlessly seeking flaws that can be eliminated or routines that can be improved. They communicate with the allies who pull for them about how and why they missed a shot. They do not kick the camera or the coach. Their careers depend on applying knowledgeable criticism and rectifying mistakes.

To shrug off the cloak of inferiority, you must find the honest critics, the friends, the mentors, the coaches who will help you refine your goals—no matter if they are personal or professional. When you can say to someone whose values you admire and judgment you trust, "Give me your advice on this—I'd really welcome any feedback," you're on the way to a whole new ballgame!

## Stop Blaming Others

The pathetic, self-destructive heroine of the recent prize-winning play *Night, Mother* informs her mother that she is planning on a neat suicide, right after giving Mother a manicure. The play is about fifteen minutes old at this point. For the remainder of the performance, we witness hysterical pleading, cajoling, bickering, joking—the whole gamut of verbal and nonverbal techniques that mothers and daughters use in dealing with each other.

Imagine the situation: Mother doesn't want her only daughter to die! She will pull every rabbit out of any hat to change her girl's mind. The daughter is miserable —she blames "life." She has no purpose. To her, life is a tattered, unappealing rag she is anxious to discard. She resents her mother, she misses her dead father, she's angry at her ex-husband, she's unable to communicate with her runaway son. She is unemployed, divorced, overweight, epileptic, terrified to venture out of the house—an agoraphobe.

Daughter Jessie is an exaggerated portrait of a woman overcome by real and imagined disabilities; her utterances about the futility of life are quite riveting for women. We've all considered every one of her arguments, though we may not have used them against ourselves all at once, as Jessie has. Jessie is a blamer. Her mother, her father, her own body, her marriage, whatever—she blames them all for failing her. She believes that ending her life is the only way to exonerate her mother, especially, and to free herself.

On a lesser, more mundane scale, we often wear a cloak of inferiority similar to Jessie's. We blame others until our last mortal breath and die either quarreling or regretful. But if we are smart cookies, we can begin to see what the real payoff is for blaming—you get no closer to what you believe others have maneuvered you out of! If that's enough of a reward for you, then clasp the cloak of inferiority closer to your bones. If it's not enough, take steps to get what you want.

Every time you find yourself pointing the finger at someone else for something that's wrong with your life—*stop*. Look closely at the situation. Is it really someone else's fault or are you just using that person as an excuse to cover up something you'd rather not face about yourself? If so, face it! That's the first step toward making a change for the better, and becoming a smart cookie.

When you give up blaming, you will recognize that there are only three things each of us owns: how we think, how we behave, and how we feel. No one else is responsible for them.

# Confront Certain Truths About Friendships

Consider Beth's predicament. She is frustrated at every turn by her friends' disapproval of her efforts to set up a business in what was once the family room of her home. Beth has chosen interior decorating as a profession—an appealing outlet, she feels, for someone with her creative energy. And I thought it seemed like a good idea when I learned of Beth's plan six months ago.

Though the responsibilities of marriage and children predominate in her life, Beth believes she needs the career in order to be "true to herself," and she did what was necessary to set up a business. Now, her friends watch as Beth's business grows. They are a little jealous, baffled, and worried about the future: will they be able to chat and laugh as easily with Beth the designer as they did with Beth their old pal?

Beth is hurt and angry on occasion because her friends are not behind her efforts. They show no interest when she talks about her clients or how she solved a design problem. "They look distracted," she told me. "They change the subject; they seem not to care at all. What burns me up is that they know what I've gone through to get here." To Beth, realizing a professional goal at all is a miracle! She is a reformed excuse-maker, someone who used every opportunity— a cranky child, an unkind remark from her husband, a favorite TV show, unwashed hair, even an outright lie— to get out of either starting or finishing a career-related task.

How can Beth deal with her friends? Must she give them up, or can she sit them down and convince these women that having a business does not exclude a warm relationship with them?

Beth is a woman who doesn't like to give anything up—least of all her long-term friendships. If you're like her, you need a practical solution to an emotionally loaded situation—lack of support from people you care about and profess to love you. Their apathy brings tears to your eyes; they make you feel *bad* for feeling good about yourself. The answer then?

Don't expect others to give you permission to tear off your cloak of inferiority and make changes in your life while they shiver deep within the layers of their own.

And you can hardly wait for friends who have an investment in maintaining the status quo to bestow blessings on your projects. This is a sensitive situation; you must understand that your friends fear losing you, while you are in despair over their abandonment. To keep these friendships, play down your need for approval of your career goals from these particular women and relate to them in ways that assure comfort for all of you. If this limits the friendships, remember the alternative. It's your choice. Know too, that as you take small steps toward your goal, you'll make new friends going in the same direction and at the same speed— friends who will cheer you on all the way.

# Have a Purpose

"Where I was born and where and how I have lived is unimportant. It is what I have done with where I have been that should be of interest." Wonderful words that extraordinary American painter Georgia O'Keeffe spoke when she was ninety years old. At ninety-six, she remains true to her philosophy, living and painting in New Mexico, still an original personality, inarguably unique.

O'Keeffe is an artist, a woman who always knew who she was. Though she may have ventured down a few branching roads early in her life, they all eventually led to the right path, and she's not veered off it since. O'Keeffe had a purpose—to look at this world and translate those perceptions and impressions through color to paper and canvas. Would that we were *all* born with monumental talents and the inner strength to express them with unflagging commitment.

Most of us aren't graced with exceptional intellectual

or artistic talents. We cannot theorize like Simone de Beauvoir, perform like Meryl Streep, hit the high notes like Joan Sutherland, or tell a joke with Joan Rivers' irreverence.

But we should still make an effort to find what suits us, to search for a purpose. This holds true for everyone. Productive work and productive love, Freud said, are the two essential ingredients in life. Without a purpose, you are at loose ends. Without a goal— whether it's as lofty as a seat on the Supreme Court or as simple as working behind the notions counter at Woolworth's—you are at the mercy of those who dole out what you need in small portions. Have a purpose and you have control of your life. A purpose can even have the power to heal wounds, as in Ellen's case.

When Ellen was twenty-five, Hank left her for another woman after three years of marriage. Divorced for nine years, Ellen spent her time being divorced *to* Hank, not *from* him. He remained a consistent and ongoing force in her life. Her fantasies were rages against him, fiery speeches telling him off. But they were just the daily flexing of a self-defeating habit. Ellen's purpose was to hate Hank. Consumed with anger for him, Ellen could not focus on any other thoughts. The payoff was misery.

When I first met Ellen, she was suffering from a financial setback. She hadn't worked in nine years, but managed to get by on alimony. And the injustice of that monthly sum, ironically enough, became Ellen's purpose. Stunned by Hank's request for a divorce, Ellen had more or less signed away property and money she could have had a share of. What could she do now? How could she change her life *now?* Could she re-channel her energy into productive activity?

Ellen went back to school and got a degree that

allows her to work in divorce mediation. "I've been through it all and I can understand what other women are feeling," she told me. Nine years passed before the emphasis on her divorce shifted from a personal context to a social one, but it happened. She's still somewhat emotionally fragile, but she's not entombed in her house with no reason to get up in the morning.

Ellen will tell you: Purpose brings you life!

## Give Up the Past

"I finally gave up the search for my father," a patient told me one afternoon, astonishing me. "Or," she amended cheerfully, "maybe I should say the need to have my father be my *idea* of a father."

Laura, just turned forty, has been fatherless for thirty-seven of her years. When her parents divorced, she was three years old. Her father subsequently demonstrated no interest in her and contacted Laura only once over the next three decades. Although he was never present in her life, she was obsessed with knowing him. Last year she made an effort to meet with him. Who, she was compelled to ask, was this man who had so forcefully shaped her life? She wanted to find out.

When Laura gave me the news about ending her search, she'd just tracked him down to a seaside town in northern California. Whom did Laura discover?

"My first response after not seeing him for so many years was, *is that all?* How I feared him! The thought that I had been rejected by my father always stirred sadness, anger, hurt and guilt in me. How would I feel now? As it turned out, I was surprisingly calm, though terrified at moments," she said.

"I saw my father as he is," Laura continued, "and

did not apologize for him. Here was a man who was ill-humored, ungiving, uncaring. He was prosperous and suspected my motives for seeing him."

Laura went back and spent time with him on four more occasions, and each encounter was less and less painful for her. "I had to accept that he did not want to be my father," Laura said. "He didn't stay away all my life out of shyness or business trips or a host of other excuses I'd created for his negligence. Fathering was not for him. And I discovered I could not make him a father now or ever."

A painful realization. A flat-out declaration of rejection from a parent is something we've all feared. That fear can be awesome. "The truth was that my father had nothing to give me," Laura concluded, "and I went back four times, each time wanting to prove he *did*. I felt sad—sad for me and sad for him. He'd not only missed out on knowing me, but also a chance to enjoy my three children, my husband, my husband's family. Yes, I feel sad, but at least I was face to face with the object of a lifelong obsession and could finally free myself from it."

Laura's search ended in disappointment on one hand (her father would not participate in her life), but satisfaction on the other (by meeting him, she could sweep her thoughts clean of fantasies about him; she knows absolutely how he really is). Laura could finally say goodbye.

Giving up the past requires a certain courage. There is no way to change what's done, and there is no way to make others conform to our dreams. Laura's father did not apologize for leaving, for not being there for her. She wanted to ask it of him, but exercised extreme restraint. Her perceptions of this man, her father, were accurate. He would not give anything. Pushing him to justify his actions would only cause her greater pain.

If it's reconciliation we seek with people in our past, then each side must be willing to compromise a little—events and conversations cannot be perfectly engineered to occur the way we rehearse them in our heads. If it's resolution of a relationship we're after, then proceed in as mature a fashion as possible. Like Laura, you may be able to declare your independence from someone who helped to wrap you in the cloak of inferiority.

Living in the past is a worthless endeavor. Dust collects at a remarkable speed. None of us can excise our histories, but we can reinterpret a past event so it has no power over us. Now's the time to do it.

# Demonstrate Competence

My hunch is that nearly every woman reaches a peak moment of doubt about her capabilities, reasoning powers, or ability to act independently, especially when a man is around. At this peak of doubt, and at every step on the craggy way up, we "forget" relevant knowledge, screw up, break down, sabotage efforts, turn down opportunities—all to assure men we still need them.

"Sometimes she made more money than her husband did; to avoid fighting about it, she would purposely lose her purse." The woman who forfeited her purse rather than give up her job or jeopardize the relationship with her husband was Betty Friedan, one of the major forces behind the women's movement. This poignant bit of Friedan's early history, reported by Marilyn French in a portrait of the feminist leader for *Esquire*, represents something millions of women have done to themselves in a multitude of different ways to protect a relationship with a man.

Why do women forgo competence? The reasons are not only personal, but are also strongly influenced by politics and economics. We can look at Friedan and her generation and pinpoint the reactionary philosophies that shaped nearly all of these women. They were raised to be "good girls," to emphasize form over feelings, to be taken care of by men. It's this "care," when it's at its most stultifying, that even now keeps women wrapped in a cloak of inferiority. The old philosophy demands that they not give up their "finest" quality—the ability to be dependent.

To demonstrate competence by accepting a promotion, founding a business, expressing ambition, or even exploring the world with only a camera and a spirit of adventure, means a woman can live without being cared for as if she were a child. Expressing competence implies a certain amount of self-sufficiency. With it comes the gratifying knowledge that you have skills, talents, and capabilities that are valued by you and by others who can benefit from your knowledge. Men can be threatened by this. They fear you won't need them once you show the world you are capable. What woman hasn't confronted her husband's resistance?

"My husband's tragedy didn't come from the fact of not understanding me," the extraordinary Golda Meir once said to Oriana Fallaci for her book *Interview With History*. "He understood me very well. It came from the fact that he *did* understand me, and at the same time realized that he couldn't change me. In short, he knew I had no choice, that I had to be what I was. But he didn't approve; that's it. And who knows if he wasn't right?"

She never doubted her place in history, but Golda Meir, committed to an ideal, always questioned who she was in the scheme of things—sometimes modestly, sometimes not. Saddened by her husband's plight in their relationship, she was who she was and devoted her energies, first, to her country.

Though I do not suggest that everyone go out and found an Israel or a women's movement or build a backyard business into a masterpiece of corporate profitmaking, I do entreat you to allow yourself a measure of competence and commitment. Each day, ask yourself: Is my life in balance? As I give to others, am I giving to myself? How can I do what I do without excluding the man in my life? When life is in balance, there will be a miraculous sense of oneself as a competent woman with a connection to productive work, enriching those connections to others.

One dilemma involving the cloak of inferiority is so enormous that I've given it space of its own—going *from no power to NO! power*. It's a dilemma we all share—believing that we are powerless, that we have no voice to be heard in this life of ours, no way to say emphatically and with larger significance, NO! I'll show you how to do it with ease.

# 3

## From No Power to NO! Power

Ruth tucks her long red hair under a wool cap, takes a deep breath, buttons her coat, then sits down on her kitchen chair. She's not sure about leaving the house. Her teenage son, her youngest, shambles through the kitchen and announces he'll be out until seven that evening. Ruth nods to him and then notices that his shoes need repair. She looks at her own boots, pivoting them by the heels. They're cracked and stained with white salt marks from two winters' wear. They make her cry. Tearily, she looks at the clock, knowing she'll be late for the appointment unless she gets up in a few minutes.

It's 1980, one day of a raw winter. All Ruth's energy goes into getting to her car; she reminds herself how to put the car in gear. The car starts; she'd hoped it wouldn't. Now she must face the doctor.

The couches are brown, like her coat. Ruth secretly thinks that maybe she'll blend in nicely and the doctor won't notice she's there. She's asked a question: Why has she come for help? Ruth rebuttons her coat, puts her hands in her pockets. Her voice sounds loud to her when she reveals that she wants out of her marriage. How long has she been married? What's wrong? Ruth begins to cry and cannot say another word. The coat is too warm.

After three sessions, Ruth begins to really speak. Twenty-two years ago she married young to a man ten years her senior. She loved him; he made her feel protected. Their three children arrived within five years. That was okay. She loved children. It was the marriage. The cause was not just her husband; it was her.

"For fifteen years we lived with my in-laws. That is, we lived with them from the second week we married," she said. "I had no territory there, few rights. I was the stranger in the household. I came last, always last. His mother came first, then his father, his brothers, his children."

Ruth begged her husband to leave his mother's house, for them to live as a family without parental influence. Will refused. With each passing year, Ruth felt more like a shadow in the household as her husband and in-laws took command. She wrote poetry, keeping it hidden. Then a journal, hidden elsewhere. One day she began to cry and couldn't stop. For three days it went on. Will, in a panic, checked her into a hospital. After six weeks she felt calmer. A nurse befriended her, encouraged her to write, to do something for herself so others wouldn't hurt her so. Then it was time to go back home to what had never been her home.

Ruth can barely remember how she summoned the courage to tell Will that if they didn't move out, she'd leave with the children. She held her ground to save her life. They moved. Free from his parents' influence,

Ruth and Will lived like traditionally married couples, but for them it was the first time. She got to know him. Will was basically a good man—hardworking, well-meaning. But he held on to Old World values. They were values that his mother affirmed, but they were not for Ruth. She wanted more, a more creative life. The children were getting older; they'd be leaving for college. What would become of her? A year later, her father-in-law died. Her mother-in-law, now alone in her house, asked them to return. Ruth refused. Two months later her mother-in-law died. Will was inconsolable, blaming Ruth for the woman's death. Will withdrew from her; Ruth became more desolate, lonely, oppressed.

This sadness brought her, that winter day in 1980, to seek help—she had had enough of sadness. She was frightened, but ready to find life at the age of forty-four before it was too late.

This gentle woman who once sat wrapped in a coat would never have predicted that in 1984 she'd be nearing the completion of a master's degree in psychology. Four years earlier, her world was a mixture of vague dreams and a tragic lack of communication. Ruth triumphed. Her marriage is still together, but it's changed, and so has her perception of it, because *she* has—and all because she knew when and how to say no to her in-laws and her husband—to exert her NO! power to save the integrity of her life.

So many of us go through our lives with no power instead of NO! power. To explain what I mean by that concept, here's a brief exercise involving a woman named Gail and a number of people in her life. As you read the statements directed at her, think about how you'd frame *your* responses.

> *Gail's friend:* Care for a chocolate? Actually, take the box home. *I'm* on a diet. Another pound won't matter on you.
>
> *Gail's mother:* Since you get up early, I don't know why you can't run a few errands for me. You can make the time.
>
> *Gail's husband:* Take that dress back to the store and no arguments. No wife of mine is wearing that.
>
> *Gail's child:* I told you to iron my gym suit for tomorrow!
>
> *Gail's neighbor:* Isn't this a coincidence meeting you and finding out you're married to Bob! I went out with him once and thought he was a total jerk.
>
> *Gail's doctor:* Take the medicine as I prescribed it and don't ask questions.

What kind of life can we assume Gail leads? Taking the statements one by one, we can theorize that the individuals in Gail's life are practiced at taking advantage or intimidating her, while she has little practice in saying no or standing up for her rights. The evidence?

A friend on a diet encourages weight increase on Gail's part and at the same time puts her down for the shape she's in. Gail's mother, demanding a favor, evinces little respect for how Gail chooses to apportion her time. Gail's husband orders her to return a dress, implying that she is not entitled to her own taste. Gail's child, like her father, shows no consideration of her feelings, but seems to think of her as a service that must function on deadline. A neighbor's insulting remark about once dating Gail's husband, Bob, implies that she thinks Gail a jerk, too. And Gail's doctor can't be bothered.

Though Gail is a fictional character, many women like her experience similar scenarios every day. Unable to say no, all their energy is channeled into making others comfortable while denying their own basic human rights as human beings with goals, sensitivities and choices. To many women, a husband's orders, a neighbor's put-downs or a parent's demands are not just brief annoyances or one-time interactions—they are ongoing reinforcement of this simple fact: The women have *no power.*

If I could define the one indicator that exclusively describes the shape of a woman's life, it would be whether she's got no power or NO! power. No power (not any power at all, or a token amount) results from a complex circuitry that most women have been wired into from an early age. Let's go back to Gail as an example. Steeped in no power, she feels obliged to be a ministering angel—putting others' needs miles before her own and at the same time taking abuse for her efforts. Because she is unable to say no, she gets herself into unnecessary binds. She is driven to apologize to the person from whom she needs information or assistance, fearing that she'll be yelled at for daring to ask for anything. Gail, of course, is not alone. Historically, women have been trained to tend to others, to be submissive and quick to follow orders, sacrificing their own needs so others may have what they, the women, believe cannot be theirs. Women are used to having no power.

"While men accept the fact that they have the ability to affect, to influence, and to change persons and social situations," note Susan M. Osborn and Dr. Gloria G. Harris in *Assertiveness Training for Women*, "many women are very reluctant to acknowledge having any power whatsoever. Like the term aggression, they reject the notion of power and any suggestion of their ability to affect change."

We are going to change that here if we can. The changes won't be made by tearing precious relationships apart, but by applying the techniques of forthrightness in a gentle but firm way.

We are going to take Gail and the millions of women who share her problem through the progression from no power to NO! power. NO! power is assertion, fairness, getting your share without depriving or hurting others. With NO! power you can make changes. The goal of NO! power is not to become like the people who strip you of power. NO! power, instead, is an *equitable balance* between you and others—based on mutual respect. NO! power is standing up for your rights without trampling on the rights of others. The final goal of NO! power is loving relationships and positive behavior patterns.

To go from no power to NO! power, a woman must recognize her own value whether or not anyone else does. She will have to forgo old habits—manipulations, game-playing, blaming others, excuses—that prevent her from developing into the best she can be. These habits are part of no power. They ensure that a woman will be indirect, coy, indecisive, deceitful.

Going from no power to NO! power involves learning how to trust your own judgment. It requires understanding of how you set up situations that guarantee losses—picking on your husband before asking him for what you want; sniping at the children so they don't cooperate and deliberately cause a greater mess; ignoring your mother for two weeks, then requesting that she take care of the kids for a weekend.

Going from no power to NO! power means that as you read through this chapter, you must examine your relationships with your children, your husband, parents, friends, neighbors. Are you treated as you treat them? Are you victimized or do you contribute to the victimization of others? As you go from no power to NO! power, you will have to figure out how your new assertiveness fits into the lives of others. You will have to be prepared for comments like "I can't believe this is the same Gail I always knew. The Gail I knew was such a sweet, good, generous girl." Or, "How dare you say no to your mother, *your mother,* at a time like this?"

There are a number of steps you will be taking to change your life, starting now. First and foremost, don't rebel alone. You need allies. I'm here for you, but find a friend, too. This friend should share your goals of becoming more assertive. You need the support of another person or group to progress, to practice the techniques, and to be nourished by the love and support that come from the solidarity of friendship.

NO! power begins here.

# Assertive Behavior Defined

Assertive behavior offers exciting possibilities if only because it represents strength, resolve and respect for yourself and others. Let's spell out some absolutes of assertion, then pose a few situations that can eventually help take you from no power to NO! power.

Assertion and aggression are not identical—do not believe any rumors to the contrary. Here's why: Assertion is like having the right of way at the wheel of a late-model Cadillac; aggression is like deliberately plowing into another car at a demolition derby. Aggression is hostile comments or jokes at another's expense; assertion means using humor to defuse a volatile situation diplomatically or to connect to another human being by a shared sense of comedy. Aggression is a disregard for the consequences of your actions; assertion involves taking responsibility. Assertion is freedom from the persistent aggravation of a recurrent problem; aggression re-creates problems. Assertion is common courtesy; aggression means pushing others around in their own lives.

Assertive behavior enables a person to stand up and act in her own best interest without excessive anxiety, fear or need for duplicity. Assertive behavior validates the assumption that you are a person worthy of respect and attention. The assertive woman can exercise personal rights without denying the rights of others. Being assertive means being able to say *no* and have others accept it. Assertion does not barrel over other people, trample on their beliefs in favor of yours, or deny them the right to disagree with you. Assertive behavior intends to be fair. And, most importantly, assertive action does not show its force by dominating others, thereby denying and diminishing their dignity.

When you are assertive, taking risks in relationships will come naturally; you can express honest feelings and opinions. If a friend insists on being an hour or more late for each appointment, how liberating it will be to say, "Marsha, unless you honor the time we agree on to meet, it's foolish for us to make appointments. I know you don't do this deliberately, but waiting wastes my time. If you can't be on time for lunch this Thursday, I know you'll understand if I leave after a few minutes." Marsha may well use this showdown to accuse you of eroding her affection, trust and understanding (part of being Marsha is being late—you knew that, didn't you?) and promise never to call you again. If she is worth your friendship, though, she will meet you halfway. This is all you can ask when you take such risks. Some responses will create comfort and harmony for you in the future; others may be shocking ("Really, how dare you!"), with cheeks coloring to a high crimson ("What happened to the nice, sweet girl I used to know?") and run-on threats, spite, bitterness, even envy.

But whatever the negative response, you will survive! And you will survive to experience the many benefits of assertive behavior.

- It will allow you to give to yourself what you'd normally and reflexively give to others—the right to express yourself as a complete person.
- It will allow you to express your curiosity because you feel freer to ask questions, take up challenges, and eliminate some of the stifling complacency you may have fallen into.
- It will give you a sense of self-worth and a high confidence level.

Assertion produces results, while nonassertion results in others creating life for us. The truth is that if we go through life giving in to the wishes of others, always holding back our own desires or even denying them, we whittle away at who we are.

When you learn to be assertive, you can exercise a number of assertion techniques at will and know when to use them and how. *Not every situation calls for an assertive response*—sometimes it's risky to speak up too firmly or too soon. Here's an important example: The woman who is locked into a marriage in which she has no economic power or emotional support is in no position to take a firm stand and leave her husband unless she has an adequate backup system. A hasty, truth-telling departure, inspired by sheer bravado, may leave her in worse condition than before. Until she can provide herself with a good fallback position, staying within the marriage is more crucial to her well-being than being "assertive"—that is, letting her husband know her true feelings about him and her desire to leave. I say this because no smart cookie would carelessly put herself in a position of being further hurt. If she cannot leave, she must protect herself until the time is right.

# Becoming Assertive

Going from no power to NO! power, then, requires the following:

- A sense of your *goals* as an assertive woman
- An *assessment* of how comfortable you are in a given setting
- *Practice* in being assertive
- *Willingness* to change your behavior
- *Keeping up your efforts* and not giving in to discouragement
- *Caring about others* and not forgetting to take care of yourself

Before reaching these milestone points to NO! power, we will no doubt encounter a few personal obstacles. These obstacles hinder our progress, keeping us from leading more productive lives. They are manifested both in what we do and in our general personality type.

# Finding Your Type

Most of us are not aggressive, passive, apologetic, indirect, oblique, fair or compassionate *all* the time, but we tend toward one type of behavior that may or may not emphasize some degree of assertion. It is this dominant personality style that describes, in part, who we are. For example, under certain circumstances even the most passive woman can stand up for herself in her own particular way. She can summon great courage and strength and display a masterfully assertive or aggressive display of temperament if her child is in danger. If there is no time to hesitate, she must act decisively. It is also possible that a generally aggressive woman known for bearing down on others or making decisions that determine the solvency of a corporation could panic and "shut down" under the similar circumstances of a child in danger. She cannot act; she's paralyzed by fear. As the situation dictates, we can react one way or the other. What gets us in trouble is favoring one style of behavior too frequently so that we don't act in our best interest. Being too passive (the Good Girl), too oblique or confusing (the Plotter) or too aggressive (the Tough Cookie) offers a number of setbacks when healthy assertion is the goal.

Let's look at the types and how they are characterized.

*The Good Girl.* As the label implies, the Good Girl

allows others to make decisions for her, all the while resenting the outcome. She expects that her life will shift by turns, each turn manipulated by others. Whether it's abrupt transition or subtle change, often she's had no say in the matter. The Good Girl, who's learned to please and pamper others as a way of life, may feel powerless, inhibited, helpless. She is most comfortable when following the directives or directions of others, fearful about being the first to take a step, state an opinion or make a change. She fears rejection, disapproval, making a mistake. The Good Girl can suffer from psychosomatic complaints such as headaches, and may use pills to help relax her. She uses illness and physical complaints to get out of doing things. Her greatest failing: an inability to say no or venture out on her own.

*The Plotter.* The Plotter secretly doubts her ability to get anything, and so becomes the mistress of trickery, deception, and, if she has the imagination and wherewithal, elaborate plots. The Plotter cannot ask for anything outright—she's indirect, denying her needs rather than letting anyone know what she wants. She fears that if others learn her desires, they will prevent her from getting them. In contrast to the Good Girl, the Plotter, coy in style, can appear deceptively assertive as she travels the circuitous path to what she wants. She may exhaust herself maneuvering her way to her goals, but that's okay with her. Games and strategies affirm that she's alive and functioning. Even her friends and family don't really trust her. Her greatest shortcomings: difficulty in making a direct statement or offering an honest opinion, and failure to get a good grasp of reality.

*The Tough Cookie.* The Tough Cookie bows to a

belief in emotional self-expression, as long as the expression is hers. She appears confident, but is actually unsure of the precarious pose she's put on display for the world. The Tough Cookie does not interest herself in the feelings of others—she is quick to humiliate others; her children and husband are not exempt from her terrorization. It's not unusual for the Tough Cookie to bully them, believing it is her right to do so. That she alienates others is a constant surprise to her. Finally, the Tough Cookie thinks that she's all right, but that the world around her is cruel, given to inconveniencing her at the most inappropriate times. Like her sister, the Good Girl, the Tough Cookie operates from the same common denominator—a sense of insecurity and a fear of disapproval. The Good Girl will bend to rules to avoid disapproval; the Plotter will find a way around them or break the rules in front of you, but feel guilty; the Tough Cookie will defy you to deny she has such vulnerability—her veneer, she hopes, is too hard to crack. The hardest thing for her: saying something positive and caring to another while desperately needing acceptance herself.

*The Assertive Woman.* Emotions exist for her in as balanced a manner as possible—she tries not to swing between extremes but to exercise self-control. She feels good about herself, can express her opinions and has little need to put others down. She doesn't look at the issue of winning or losing, but tries to reach some conciliatory position. She struggles with the Good Girl, the Plotter and the Tough Cookie aspects of herself. The Assertive Woman is you, me and any other woman of any color or shape. She is a composite of qualities— compassionate and nurturing; she can open a door for someone or graciously thank the person opening a door for her. She can be dependent on a man or live independent of any immediate family. She can be soft-spoken and loving, yet stand up for her principles. She has available to her the greatest, most extensive choices of who to be.

Suppose that four women get together to socialize casually. This could be a familiar situation in your life—you, a close friend, your sister, her sister-in-law, are having lunch at a coffee shop. For argument's sake, let's imagine that each woman represents one distinct type on the assertiveness scale. (It might be more accurate at times that four Good Girls meet, or that the group is dominated by Plotters. No matter. What we want to see clearly is how conclusions are formed as *each* type reacts in relation to the others and expresses herself. This, truly, is real life.)

Imagine, then, that the news has just reached this group that a fifth friend hàs announced an upcoming marriage to a man she's known only for a month. The friend, thirty-five years old and childless, has been married once before. The man she's marrying, divorced with custody of two teenage children, is forty-eight. The conversation opens:

*The Assertive Woman:* I think Harry will be good for Sue. She says she really likes his kids, too. What could be better?

*The Good Girl:* You're probably right, but I hear her mother is upset because they're not having a big wedding. How can she do that to her own mother?

*The Tough Cookie:* Give me a break with the wedding! Personally, I think Sue's crazy for marrying that man. Who wants to deal with *two* bratty kids at her age? Someone should tell Sue that being a stepmother is tantamount to suicide! Those kids'll kill her. This marriage will never work. Don't think I won't warn her.

*The Plotter:* I think Harry just wants to marry Sue so he'll have someone to take care of his kids.

*The Assertive Woman:* What do you mean? That Harry is not really in love with Sue?

*The Plotter:* Harry's interesting . . . real slick, if you know what I mean. . . .

*The Good Girl:* You're always so clever about people!

*The Tough Cookie:* I think Sue must be *desperate.*

*The Assertive Woman:* It doesn't matter if we think she's desperate or not. Look at Sue—she's so *happy.*

*The Tough Cookie:* Even if Sue asks me, I may not go to her wedding just to show her what I think of her decision.

*The Assertive Woman:* Waitress! We'll have the check, please.

# Examining the Obstacles to NO! Power

A new patient tells me that she's been living with a man who, she discovered to her horror, has been stealing from her. She's bound by sex to Pete—he's a superb lover, Donna insists, a man who *moves* her as no other could. But essentially he's a crook. To leave him, she ran off to Illinois to stay with her ex-husband, who welcomed her back. She loves her ex-husband, Donna says, but sex with him wasn't and isn't as potent a force as with Pete. Now she's back in Detroit, not knowing what to do. Her thieving lover wants her back; he alternately begs and threatens her daily. "What can I do?" Donna cries. It's so hard to say no (that is, NO!) to Pete, to know that she may have to give him up.

Upon questioning Donna I uncover Pete's attitudes: He tells Donna that she's selfish for leaving, not to mention niggling and unforgiving over the money. "So what about the money?" he asks sanctimoniously. "You've got it!"

Donna talks easily about the situation, asks for advice and comfort. But what's missing here is the *N* factor, a trait absent in many women like her. Donna does not know how to defend herself and say NO! because she's tripping over a few obstacles. She thinks that this must be the course of her life (the myth that personal history is irreversible) and that she must automatically put others' needs first (the myth that compassion shows you're a real woman). Above all, she doesn't know why she keeps going back for more.

Donna would agree that it's normal for Pete to take advantage of her—she's a woman, Pete's a man, and what more explanation does anyone need! As with many women who are abused by others, she permits the status quo—continuing to make things agreeable for others, not for herself—while feeling powerless to back down.

So, Pete wants something from her—her money, her body and her life—and what matters to both Donna and Pete is Pete's desire. In truth, Donna wants Pete to change his basic character so as to be a different *kind* of man, but not to change his role as her perfect lover with whom she can abandon herself. What she'd prefer is to take the desirable characteristics of both her husband and her lover and combine them into one ideal man.

Meanwhile, she faces obstacles to gaining NO! power. Let's see how they and other traps like them work to stop *you*.

# Personal History

Except for the one or two rare examples of human perfection who have lived lives graced with complete acceptance, love, respect and support of their achievements by others, people *everywhere* have been hurt, have failed and have suffered crises of confidence. Each of us who has walked this earth can remember that moment—or even recount hundreds of moments—when we've been felled by an emotional plague, gone down for the count, feverish and cursing. We remember how, after the tears had dried, how hurt, disappointed and disillusioned we felt, and are surprised that we survived the onslaught. As a result of each unpleasant moment, a negative thought may have been reinforced. You set out on a quest and failed; your family celebrates your failure and reminds you that you've *always* been someone who "couldn't finish what you started." The man you love leaves you for another woman. To make sure it never happens again, you marry the man you wouldn't even date five years earlier because he's available (nowhere near your equal), a man you're sure of.

When you transform past history into today's excuses for not becoming a woman who fights for her dignity, you go nowhere and gain nothing. "If I could only figure out why my mother didn't love me, why my father was so vain and uncaring, why I wasn't born into a privileged family and why I feel so powerless because I'm poor and always will be," are some of the many forms of questioning the past. "If I knew," goes the conjecture, "then I'd be able to stand up for myself."

The questions persist. We torture ourselves with such inner harassment, falsely convinced that we cannot have what we have not had so far!

You may never figure out where it all started, and, honestly, it doesn't matter. Yesterday no longer exists, so why make it larger than life today, letting old images swallow up the time you have. If you are ready to accept responsibility for who you are and who you want to be, if you can make a decision that you want to change, you will. And you can start by cutting loose those parts of yesterday that keep you back.

# Fear of Making Mistakes

"Remember," Stanlee Phelps and Nancy Austin advise sagely in their fine book *The Assertive Woman*, *"that to be assertive does not mean to be perfect"* (my italics). Those who are unable to function or take a first step because they believe perfection will elude them, please take heed. Perfection is not your goal. Growth is your goal, and mistakes are critical to getting there.

The toddler learning how to use a fork doesn't feel like a fool when the food drops between lift-off from the plate and his mouth. Nor does he abuse his own efforts by saying, "You're looking at an incompetent eighteen-month-old who can't handle a simple tool like a three-tined fork. Give up on me from now on." The child is unselfconscious as he acquires skills. He learns to stand, walk, talk, crack the code to the childproof lock and find his place at the table with civilized manners by making mistakes and correcting them.

To go from no power to NO! power, allow yourself some of that early joyous discovery of life. If you make a mistake, acknowledge it with good humor and set about to learn more. Most mistakes are not catastrophic, life-changing or irreparable. Acknowledge them and move on.

# The Put-Down

Your husband watches you walk toward him across the living room and flashes a look of extreme dissatisfaction or irritation. You ask what's wrong and he denies expressing any "look" at all. That discomfort stays with you. You run into an old school chum when you're with your handsome new husband and the next day she calls with the dig: "How did someone who looks like you get someone who looks like him!" You're sitting with four other people in a coffee shop and you ask the waitress for coffee spoons. She distributes spoons to everyone and leaves you out; you're obliged to ask again. Still you feel obliged to leave a fifteen-percent tip.

Why do put-downs have such a devastating effect on us? The put-down may have a small element of truth to it, but its force tends to be directed more toward clobbering you than helping you with legitimate criticism. Put-downs are delivered out of envy, frustration, hostility, mistrust of others, defensiveness, or maybe you're just providing free material for someone's jokes. Sometimes you are the target of the put-down, other times you just happen to be standing in the line of fire when the gun goes off.

How should you handle the put-downs as mentioned here? You can ask your husband what's bothering him, and if he says, "Nothing," let him know you're aware it's "something," but it's his decision to tell you or not. To your chum, merely reply to her appraisal of your looks as cheerfully as possible. "So nice hearing from you again, Trudy, but I have to run." And hang up! As for the waitress, a tip rewards service; it's really not an obligation. Poor service? No tip.

Know, too, that not every put-down need be taken personally or answered at all. As you become more assertive, you will be able to distinguish between those incidents that require protecting yourself and those that don't. Most of all, fear of the put-down need not be an obstacle to personal growth.

## Oh! I'm Sorry

How often do you say, "I'm sorry," for deeds you never committed or as an automatic two-word introduction to any request or statement of intention you make? Do you persist in apologizing when you want to say no? At least once in her life *every* woman has said, in effect, "Hello, I'm sorry," while being totally innocent of any blame. I still have to fight from doing this, too.

If saying you're sorry and therefore feeling guilty has become an obstacle to assertive behavior, *listen* to when those two little words tumble from your lips. Note those incidents. Are you apologizing for saying no when you do not want to do what others have requested or planned for you? Has a friend begged for an honest opinion and you've opened with, "I'm sorry, but—"? Did you find the courage to ask for a raise and when the boss didn't come through, make another attempt by introducing the subject with, "I'm sorry to trouble you again, but—"? Were you the one to timidly say, "I'm sorry," when *you* were rejected?

Let's discuss two common situations where women implicate themselves in apologetic behavior. In the first case, a woman is being told what she can and cannot do by her husband; in the second, she is unable to veto a request, choosing instead to be excessively polite.

## The Class: Losing Position

*Woman:* I thought I'd take a class one night a week.

*Husband:* (decisively) No, you're not.

*Woman:* (coming from the extreme end of a weak position) I'm *sorry*, but I need to get out of the house once a week.

*Husband:* You can stay home. We don't have the money to waste on school.

*Woman:* It's just one night. I promise I'll come straight home after class.

*Husband:* You're coming straight home from nowhere. You don't need school. I like you the way you are.

*Woman:* (shrilly) I'm sorry! I want that class. You have no right—

*Husband:* I told you what I think and I don't want to say it again.

This wife can battle her husband about going to school until she finally gives up. Her arguments remain weak, defensive. Let's look at the winning position now.

## The Class: Winning Position

*Woman:* Larry, I've signed up for a class once a week.

*Husband:* I don't want you taking classes.

*Woman:* What's your objection?

*Husband:* You don't need to go to school.

*Woman:* I'm not asking permission to take the class, Larry. I've already signed up and it starts on Monday.

*Husband:* I don't know why you need it. You have enough to do at home.

*Woman:* You'll see that things at home will pretty much stay the same. I'll be happy to prepare dinner beforehand and you can just warm it up.

## The Loan: Losing Position

*Borrower:* Lend me fifty dollars for a week, will you?

*Woman:* I'm sorry. I don't have the money on me.

*Borrower:* Maybe I can come by tomorrow around ten.

*Woman:* Well, I may need it to pay the fuel man.

*Borrower:* He can wait. I always pay that bill last.

*Woman:* I don't know. I also have the dentist bill.

*Borrower:* But I really need that money!

*Woman:* I'm sorry, my husband wouldn't like it . . .

You can see the outcome of this "touch." The exchange could go on until the woman writes out a check, handing over the money she can't spare. While apologizing, the woman proffers countless excuses to the person making the request, who is relentless in knocking down her arguments. The assertive solution?

# The Loan: Winning Position

*Borrower:* Lend me fifty dollars for a week, will you?

*Woman:* No, I'm not in a position to lend you money.

*Borrower:* Fifty dollars isn't much for you. Come on. Be a sport.

*Woman:* I know you want the money, but I've given it some thought and decided that it's not a good idea.

*Borrower:* Well, how about—

*Woman:* No.

When you apologize to others for your decisions, you are simultaneously telling them that you aren't worthy of having the ability to make decisions. You are also asking others to approve of your decisions and give you permission. To stop saying, "I'm sorry," out loud, you may have to start out by saying it silently to yourself.

Let others hear only the assertive statements that will follow. That's a good start.

# Taking Criticism

The major function of criticism is to consider the merits and demerits of its object, whether an act, a remark or a work of art. We think of criticism as stressing faults, as damning the person along with the characteristic that's been judged faulty, weak, unworthy, unattractive, misdirected or whatever. In reality, constructive criticism can point the way to freedom. More to the point of daily living: It is impossible to please everyone all the time, and sometimes we just need to accept those occasions when we are criticized or rejected.

Predictably, the nonassertive woman collides with the critique and feels bruised by the critic. For some women, not giving criticism to others is an assured and effective way, they believe, to avoid being criticized. But criticism need not be thought of as a form of brutality.

What makes criticism difficult for women to deal with are the elements of surprise and rejection. A boyfriend in a rocky relationship recites a list of your imperfections, from the set of your hair to the gloss of your toenail polish; you can do no right. You panic. He's never been so quarrelsome and critical before. Or, you call your husband at the office, hoping to initiate a romantic evening later, but he's abrupt, chews you out for calling, makes you feel totally foolish, then hangs up. Or, your neighbor comments on the condition of your backyard and how you might pay more attention to clipping hedges and clearing away debris. When you are vulnerable to criticism and fear rejection, the words uttered by others become ominous, significant, eloquent appraisals of, you think, *all* your inadequacies.

When you become more assertive, you are able to differentiate between the valid, constructive critique and the unrealistic, manipulative, sometimes unconscious critique that's intended to keep you off guard and unsure of yourself.

Since none of us is perfect, all of us will make mistakes, and we must be prepared to take criticism. If a critic points out a flaw or a fault, examine the contention. Does it ring true? Can you admit to that fault and begin taking steps to lessen it? If someone criticizes you for something you haven't done, or is in a gloomy mood that day, can you brush it off without emotional outbursts?

As you become more assertive, you will be able to give criticism more gracefully and in a caring way so people will seek you out for your opinion. You will also be able to look at your faults and acknowledge them openly. When you do, you will rid yourself of feeling hurt or rejected as a human being when someone else points them out.

## The Compassion Trap

One of the more eloquent descriptions of a universal obstacle to assertion was defined by writer Margaret Adams: she called it the "compassion trap," and women are especially vulnerable to it. The compassion trap results in a life devoted to serving others; making others comfortable; providing tenderness at any cost;

ensuring that men feel right and good in whatever roles they choose, even self-destructive ones; giving up cherished ambitions to help others fulfill themselves. All this sounds noble and altruistic, and it is—within reason. But remember, *it's still a trap*.

Here's why. The danger of the compassion trap is that you link your emotions exclusively to the soothing of others while you sacrifice something of yourself. If you can only look outward while others accomplish goals *for* you, your pleasure will be vicarious. It has to be, since you are an accomplice in the plot to keep you tied to someone else's ambitions. You put others before you; they are often quite happy to move forward and leave you behind.

A woman called recently and told me a story that illustrates the intensity and power of this trap. Laurie and her husband moved into her parents' home when her husband lost his job; they agreed to contribute some money to the household each week. The sum was considerably less than what they'd have needed for their own place. Six months later, Laurie's husband found a job and told her mother they'd be moving out. Mother responded with rage; she wouldn't hear of it. How dare Laurie and her husband leave when they knew she *needed* the income from their weekly contribution? The couple succumbed to her mother's fury and emotional blackmail, and are still living, unhappily, at the mercy of her parents' demands.

The compassion trap need not be home-based. Significant problems arise in business, too. We all recognize the woman who stays at a dead-end job because the boss assures her, "No one could take your place." The compliment becomes compelling—she's needed, irreplaceable. But she's also getting nowhere or working for less than what her ability is worth, and she is made to feel traitorous and guilty for wanting to leave. Or perhaps she's asked to "help out" on weekends for no pay—and no complaints about it either. Or what about the woman who refuses a promotion so that someone with "more ambition," the very person she's trained, can take the slot above her?

Within relationships, the compassion trap snaps shut with a resounding clang and assumes control. The woman who keeps finding excuses for her boyfriend's not wanting to commit to marriage ("He's not quite sure of himself yet, but I have faith in him") or the wife who blames job pressures and alcohol for her husband's habitually punishing behavior ("He's too sensitive— he's just not himself after a few drinks") are two poignant examples.

There are many components to the compassion trap that serve to keep women the experts on others' feelings and care. A woman's strength can be that very compassionate giving, caring and tending. Pursued to an extreme degree, where all her energy is poured into self-sacrifice, it may be a cushioned trap, but a trap nevertheless.

# How Assertive Are You?—Put It in Writing

A patient described an experience to me that sets the record for taking it on the chin when she should have gotten a kiss on the cheek. The episode represents Penny's particular conflict about being used by others, and shows how her assertive impulses became displaced by those of the "Good Girl." You'll see what I mean as the following story unfolds.

A close friend asked Penny for the loan of her sewing machine. Since Rita's little boy was ill at the time, Penny cheerfully taxied the machine over. The three-mile ride north to her friend's house was inconveniently out of her way on that particular day—she had errands to run in the opposite direction—but she decided to be a pal and help Rita out.

When Rita had the machine about six weeks, Penny asked for it back. Rita pleaded with Penny to let her keep it another few days to make kitchen curtains. Penny reluctantly agreed. After four more months of delay and attempts to get the machine from her friend, Penny became agitated and told Rita she had to have it back—after all, almost six *months* had passed. Annoyed, Rita demanded that Penny pick it up before noon the following day. In response Penny asked Rita to return it to *her;* after all, she borrowed it!

Rita snapped that she wasn't about to debate the issue of manners. If Penny wanted the machine, "Come over and get it!"

Penny was furious. She'd been inconvenienced for almost six months, had done her friend a good turn by hauling the machine over, and now, in payment, Rita was begrudgingly surrendering the machine and demanding Penny retrieve it herself. The world being what it was for Penny, she drove the three miles to her friend's house, feeling agitated, put upon and tearful.

At Rita's, she says, she was "suckered into a few cups of coffee. I didn't want to go along somehow giving Rita endless compliments about her none-too-terrific handiwork, but I did. Then I was made to feel bad because I was leaving with my machine. I sat there, feeling a little numb, knowing in some part of me that I should be telling Rita what I thought about her kidnapping my machine, but as usual I clicked into being Rita's great, good friend—the doormat who even travels for an insult! It was easier!"

If we surveyed Penny's life, we'd uncover a consistent pattern of "Good Girl" behavior that's self-perpetuating with a minimum of help from others. As a "doormat," Penny is conflicted about expressing her feelings, standing her ground, asking for her rights while having others respect them, and, finally, saying no. Notice something in this story that's critical to Penny's changing into a considerably more self-respecting woman? In it, she's *aware* of turning off the impulse to tell Rita that their friendship has not been honored but abused. So there is hope for Penny. But, as an impartial observer, can you clearly see how she gets herself into these situations because she needs to be a pleaser? Are your patterns similar to hers? And how about Rita? Do you identify with her, or at least know when you demonstrate such aggressive, "Tough Cookie" behavior?

Apart from the lessons in this story, the important point is that, like Penny, you want to become attuned to the true manner of your assertive behavior. Interaction with others is a topic you think about all the time. This is inevitable. Unfortunately, personal growth is not inevitable. Our capacity for growth is enormous, but it's not a biological reflex like blinking when the lights suddenly go on. It takes a concentrated effort, an expenditure of energy, and a *written chronicle* of when and how it happens.

We have tons of facts, opinions and feelings stored in our heads, and sometimes it all becomes a jumble. We forget what we can do and emphasize what we can't— we act the "Good Girl." We forget that others have feelings, so afraid are we of being deprived of one thing or another.

With a log—just an inexpensive notebook you will devote to the reporting of your actions—you will have the opportunity to examine how you behave and how you *think* you behave. Some actions will help you see in which situations you are too passive or too indirect, like Penny, or too overbearing, like Rita. Others will clarify the problems you face, the attitudes you assume, the behavior you demonstrate, the result of that behavior, and how you might have done things differently.

The idea that you will be keeping a written record of your behavior will help you stay aware of when you are positively assertive. Set up your log in the following way: At the top of a page write in the area of conflict about standing up for yourself: *Why am I afraid to confront a husband, friend, parent, boss?* Allow one page for each area of conflict, or enough space to answer these questions:

- What is my attitude about facing the situation?
- How do I typically behave?
- What am I afraid of that stops me from standing up for myself?
- What might I have done *after the fact* to let others know how I felt?
- What will I do the next time this comes up?

Write down the questions, answer them, and date the page. In one month, reread the questions and answers and see how you've progressed. Now answer *these* questions:

• Which person in particular intimidates you so that you become docile, indirect or aggressive? (Your husband, friend, parents, boss, child?)

• Do you notice the circumstances that can trigger panic, rage or irritation within you? (When someone asks for money, a favor, work without pay, an honest opinion, sex?)

• Are there questions about your personal life that you respond to with hesitation, fear or aggression? (What you've done with your life, your feelings about parents, race, religion, your age, when someone else gets the compliments?)

• Are there situations involving other people that arouse feelings of insecurity, doubt or fear? (Large parties, going for a job interview, blind dates, family reunions?)

# Changing Your Behavior

Thoughts and actions will work in tandem as you begin to change to a more assertive person. Some of you will change by thinking first and then following up with action; others will act first with a positive show of effectiveness and then change your thinking. Freudians say that you must first change your attitude and then you can change your behavior. Behaviorists say that you can *act* first (initiate a change of behavior) and *then* change your attitude. I say, do whichever works best for you. Here's what I mean: You may have always believed that swimming would be fun, but you're a little afraid of the water. Now you are determined to swim. Before you put a toe in the pool and get your first lesson, you click into a mindset that says, "Swimming's okay. I'll be safe here on the shallow end of the pool with an instructor. I will do my best to learn how to swim." You repeat this over and over again until you can do it. (Positive thoughts first, action follows.)

The alternative is to know that you'll never get over the fear of water by staying out of the pool. You decide to take action and learn how to swim. You sign up for lessons, get into the pool and think, "So far so good!" Your instructor holds on to you as you float and you hear yourself saying, "I'm okay." (Action first, positive thought follows.)

You can see how either type prepares the way for change. The point is that *both* would-be swimmers will get into the pool.

To change from no power to NO! power, you will be thinking and acting through a number of critical steps. First, you'll figure out what specific behavior you intend to change. After *identifying your goal,* you can build a progression of assertiveness-training steps, selecting the ones that work best for your success.

When you start changing behavior, don't tackle problems that are too difficult or complex. Choose simple goals that may immediately reward your efforts. The idea is not to just make points by being assertive, but to *effectively* make your point.

Let's look at some of the techniques you can use to examine and begin changing your behavior.

## Identify Triggers

Take a look at situations that set you off. What makes you passive, withdrawn, devious, angry, pushy, demanding? Do people use guilt-producing statements to get their way with you? ("If you had been here on time, I wouldn't have cut my finger slicing the potatoes for dinner!") Does someone accuse you of disappointing him even though it is possible that he sabotaged your efforts so that you were bound to fail both him and you? Are you unable to bear teasing about your weight, height, religion, hometown, race, personal style? Examine your vulnerabilities—these are the triggers that people use to get you to say yes when you want to say no.

# Body Language

Two truths: (1) Keys to assertion are directness, honesty and tact and (2) Assertion is a *skill* to be learned, not a quality we're born with like long legs. Now a third: One of the difficult aspects of assertion to understand is the power of body language. Think about the shape of a seductive pose. It's not only a matter of revealing clothing, but also how the body tips forward, how one projects a yielding look through posture and facial expression. You know the physical look, too, of the "stone maiden," the ungiving woman. She's all stiff posture, hands folded in her lap, head tipped slightly back, and a contemptuous air about her.

Just as a woman should learn to move with a certain energetic grace, so should she extend that grace to *assertive posture.* Can you imagine giving a raise to a woman who clumps into your office, flops into a chair, and intones in a whiny voice that she deserves a raise—either barely glancing at you or staring you down? Other distracting, unattractive and counterproductive gestures of the "clumper" are hair-twirling, moving eyebrows at a rapid pace, chain-smoking, gum-cracking, picking at clothes or fingers, standing with hunched shoulders or with weight on one foot. Each gesture or stance signals a message to others which says, "I'm not at my best, but I have come to you to ask for more, anyway."

Here's where a full-length mirror and a friend with a superbly critical eye can help. With her or him, you will rehearse how to look and sound when making a request or stating an opinion that matters in your scheme of things. You should stand straight, shoulders back. Get feedback from this trusted friend on how you look before you face the real thing. Be sure that facial expressions match what you will be saying, and don't exaggerate the mood. Do not grimace as if in pain when you tell the boss you are unhappy about the work schedule. Your boss will get the point without any accompanying childish facial gestures; (s)he will respect you more without them. When you confront your husband with the news that you'd like him home for dinner before nine o'clock at least twice a week, don't smile sweetly and speak your message as though it were a question, thereby lessening the impact of a serious request. Be aware of what you can't see about yourself by asking others to tell you. Then practice controlling the habits or tics that are sabotaging your efforts.

How did you sound when you said what you meant? Was there a whininess to the request? ("Oh, come *on*, Greg—you *never* let me have it my way.") Were you shrill when bringing up a bone of contention? ("We'll see who's going where on Saturday night!") Did you stutter, mumble, sound choked up with tears?

The voice is a miraculous and versatile instrument.

We can change the meaning of words subtly by intonation. A simple phrase like "I must say no, thank you" can take on a universe of meanings depending on how it's sent. It can be spat out harshly, made to sound sarcastic by stressing "thank you," turned into an aggressive directive by allowing a beat between words and keeping the sound at a monotone, or said quietly, as if it's a vague idea. The assertive voice? Unless you sound positive, upbeat and direct, you may allow others to manipulate you into a change of heart, an argument, or whatever typical result you are trying to change. To help you solve the problem, get a tape recorder. Once you are aware of how you sound when you practice speeches, you can improve delivery, speak to others decisively and eventually gain power.

## Listen to Others

Do you find yourself distracted when others speak? Do you ask others to repeat themselves? Are you interested in what others have to say? *This is important:* Always allow others to make a statement, listen to what's actually said, and infer what's left unsaid. You will realize that people may come on very strongly, but underneath they are hesitant, unsure. As part of assertiveness training, listen to others. Take a beat before you respond—don't start replying until the speaker has finished her or his piece. We can get ourselves into trouble by tuning out others' feelings and thoughts, finishing others' sentences or interrupting before they've completed what they were going to say. That gives the speaker an opportunity to say, "I never was going to say that in the first place. That's the trouble with you, you're always second-guessing me. *I* would have said—" The result: You will have to apologize. Avoid apology—pay attention to others!

## Practice Positive Self-Talk

When's the last time you said something complimentary to someone? Just a few hours ago? When's the last time you said something flattering about yourself? Months ago—and meekly? Self-acknowledging behavior is a tough problem for many people. We're not usually encouraged to speak of our own finer qualities —we're afraid people will think we're conceited, grandiose, self-inflated. Shirley MacLaine accepted her Oscar for *Terms of Endearment* and said, proudly and with the kind of courage that brings applause, "Thank you. I earned it." Can you feel positively toward people like Shirley MacLaine who commend themselves when they achieve a goal? Could you say, "Thank you, I earned it," *out loud* with dignity and not a gloating pride?

What's said out loud begins inside—self-talk. Self-talk is simple and produces brilliant results. When people think about getting power or making changes, they ruminate about it—it's all images, words, unstructured incidents tumbling around in their head. This is inner dialogue—self-talk. Self-talk is decisive. People with no power tell themselves they have no power. ("This is beyond me." "I'll never get anywhere." "He's all I could get." "I'll never be hired for that job.") Belief in yourself—*faith* in yourself and what you can accomplish—begins with positive self-talk.

# Taking a Compliment

The assertive woman regards a compliment as a simple expression of appreciation. But most women don't react well to compliments for two critical reasons.

First, since compliments may be used indiscriminately to manipulate others, we conclude that others must be using the compliments they pay us to manipulate us and discount what we're experiencing. We're often trained from early girlhood to use compliments to cheer others up ("With your personality, you'll meet another man in a minute"), to cover up inadequacy ("Your boss doesn't understand that you're not slow, Arthur, just careful"), or cool down a potentially explosive situation ("Oh, now, Helen. You're much too smart and sensitive to call his ex-wife and force a showdown. You'll see, he really loves you!"). Since our own compliments stroke egos, we wonder if we should accept others' flattery as truth or as superficial and false commentary. So, we ask ourselves, is there an ulterior motive behind the compliment? ("Why does she say I look thinner when I've just told her I gained five pounds?") Do you really look thinner that day in that dress or is it just convenient for your pal to have you believe it's so?

The other reason that women don't react well to compliments is that they are programmed to feel undeserving. Because too many of us were brought up with more negative criticism than positive affirmation, eventually the compliment, when it comes, strikes us as shocking, untrue. Having little experience with positive statements from others, we almost automatically disbelieve them. "Don't listen to that," our inner voice may say. "It can't be true." Therefore, we do not say thank you with a smile, but contradict the compliment or deny it. "You look terrific in green," a friend says, and you reply, "I thought it made my skin look too sallow." A stranger sitting next to you on the bus asks the name of your perfume and you say, "Oh, it's just some cheap stuff from the drugstore, but I like it sweet." A neighbor comments on how beautifully your quilt turned out and you parry with, "If you look closely, you can see how really botched up it is in places."

We all like flattery. We all like reassuring comments —that we look attractive (after making the effort), that we did a good job (after putting in even more effort), that we're good company (we really do care about the person we're with), or whatever else others acknowledge us for in a positive light. We need to learn how to compliment others honestly—without denying them positive feelings or being excessively unctuous about it. Most important, let's allow people to risk saying something nice to us without being put down for it.

The response to a compliment is, "Thank you."

# Don't Just Get Mad, Try a Little Creative Revenge

The fine art of creative revenge takes a number of interesting forms. In fact, the forms are limited only by your imagination. Creative revenge, to put it simply, allows you to get even—to extract some satisfactory justice—when you are wronged, but lets you do it with a sense of humor, not boiling malice. Creative revenge gives you NO! power.

## SMART COOKIES DON'T CRUMBLE

Creative revenge is not madness unreined, or tormented obsession over how to get back at a lost love, a hateful relative or a traitorous friend. Creative revenge does not require a passing knowledge of the black arts—no potions, incantations or ceremonies here. Creative revenge is not blood revenge or fury let loose. The only weapons you will use are your wits. With creative revenge, you will not avenge yourself with cruel or irrational acts toward the person (or persons) who hurt you. You will be a smart, a very smart and assertive cookie.

Creative revenge can loosen the ties that bind you to those you dislike intensely and thereby loosen the power they hold over you. And you *are* bound to those who sometimes make you delirious as you plot to get even. These people take up your time, your thoughts and your emotional energy, which would all be better spent on more productive and rewarding relationships. Creative revenge can help you excise from your life both the fury and those who've made you furious.

Here's Karen's story. It will help you understand how creative revenge works and why she felt vindicated.

One evening last spring, Karen came home from the supermarket, prepared dinner and waited for her husband, Joe, to get home. A week later she was still waiting. Joe, it seemed, had quit work, packed a few things and left. Gone without a trace. No note to Karen. No phone call. And no one knew where he was. Shattered, left with two small children and no job, she went through agonies putting her life in some sort of order. A year later to the day, Karen received a phone call from Joe.

"I'm really lonely," he told her. "I've been sailing around the world as part of a crew on a yacht, but it's not working out." Karen listened attentively. Joe continued: "I really miss home now," he told her earnestly. "I really miss that affection and a nice, warm body."

Composed, Karen asked Joe for his address. She promised he'd be hearing from her. A week later, Joe got his wish—a remembrance of home and a nice, warm body. Karen had shipped his dog to him with a note that said, "Curs of a feather."

Creative revenge has built into it a nonlethal form of punishment that puts a tormenter in his (or her) place. You make your point and make sure you don't get hurt by any boomeranging consequences of your acts. More lethal revenge often *does* boomerang: meanness begets meanness as violence begets violence. But creative revenge gives you freedom and self-esteem—you stand up for yourself without really attacking the other person. After all, you're just allowing the other person to experience the standard he or she set for you.

Franny is another woman who applied the laws of creative revenge and gained NO! power with a boyfriend who was less than kind about breaking off their relationship. She'd been living with Ben at his apartment for about three years when he told her one morning that he'd like her to move out. Since he was leaving the following morning for a three-week business trip, he told her to please be gone before he returned. And off Ben went.

For three weeks Ben was haunted by what Franny would do. He felt guilty about his insensitivity in breaking off the relationship, and knew Franny well enough to expect some reaction from her. But what? Would the apartment be devastated when he returned? Would she have shredded the sheets, smashed the dishes, done something inordinately wild to get even?

Gingerly, Ben opened the door to his apartment

three weeks later. The apartment was still neat. The lights were out. He turned them on. Everything was perfect. The same with the bedroom. Nothing unusual in the kitchen either. Then he heard what sounded like a ticking . . . no! a clicking. Had Franny planted a bomb in the dishwasher? He soon found the source. The phone was off the hook. As he lifted it to put it back in the cradle, he heard a voice. He put the receiver to his ear to hear someone telling the time. Only it wasn't the time in Chicago, his hometown. Franny had dialed the number for the time in Tokyo three weeks before and left the phone off the hook. Every ten seconds a Japanese voice uttered the time to Ben's empty kitchen.

A week later Ben received the phone bill. It only cost him a few thousand dollars for the service.

With creative revenge, you can zap the other person and leave him or her be forevermore, or make use of the incident to help re-create the relationship. Creative revenge helps you make your point; perhaps now you and the "victim" can make peace, since your feelings have been expressed in no uncertain terms. If there's still something between you, both of you may be ready to start again. Barbara, for one, tried her hand at creative revenge, and its result, ultimately, was reconciliation with a straying husband. Here's what happened.

One afternoon when Barbara got into her car, it wouldn't start. Since her husband was at a neighbor's watching a football game, she decided to take his car. She got in the driver's seat and saw his raincoat folded neatly over a few boxes on the passenger side. Lifting the coat, she discovered two gift-wrapped packages. It wasn't her birthday or their anniversary—in fact it wasn't the birthday or anniversary of anyone she could think of. Heart pounding, she ran back into the house for scissors and Scotch tape, got back into the car and took off.

Parked in the shopping mall lot, she carefully unwrapped the gifts. Inside one box was a white cashmere cardigan, and in the other, a costly gold watch.

Barbara neatly clipped all the pearl buttons off the cardigan, leaving the threads, and pried open the watch case and removed the mechanism. With shaking hands, she repacked the boxes as they were and put them back under her husband's raincoat.

For two weeks Barbara said nothing and tried to be cool while she waited for a reaction. When was Lou going to present those gifts to his girlfriend? A day later, Lou arrived home late and didn't say hello, but opened with this question: "I understand why you cut the buttons off the sweater, but why did you take the works out of the watch?"

Barbara answered without missing a beat, "I figured she'd been getting the works from you for months, anyway."

Lou laughed in spite of himself and sat down next to her. Barbara continued in a different tone: "And now that she's opened the packages, let's open the conversation. What do you want to do about *us?*"

And finally, here's Cara's story—a story which proves that to be effective, creative revenge can require little more than a quick wit.

For most of their ten-year marriage, Cara's husband, Jack, would toss insulting remarks at her about her cooking—but only at dinners with his family. Jack thought Cara's cooking skills were always good for a laugh—whether or not his observations were true didn't much matter to him. The point was to tease her unmercifully. Time and again, she asked him to stop—

his remarks sure weren't funny to her, just irritating and demeaning.

Thanksgiving came. Cara worked for days to prepare the feast for his entire family—parents, six brothers and sisters and their children. She thought she'd done a splendid job. This dinner, she thought, would finally silence Jack. He'd have to love it. But after two courses, Jack went at her again: "Cara's a great kid, isn't she?" he said, preparing her for the compliment she believed would finally tumble from his lips. "But what a lousy cook!"

Without even looking at him, Cara reached over casually for a roll and said loudly, clearly and sweetly, "Tell you what, Jack. I'll work on my cooking and you work on your lovemaking!"

There are two basic lessons to be learned in this book: (1) How to develop the attitude that you have the right to personal power and NO! power and the right to use either at will and (2) How to get and keep personal power. Power is many things—money, authority, access to what one desires—but most often in *your* life it will be a simple act like choosing what to do. ("Yes, I'm ready." "NO, I don't choose to do that.") Personal power and NO! power endow you with a sense of worth, a purpose, a feeling that you are significant, a sense that people respect you—which, on occasion, may be more important than the knowledge that they love you.

When you start to seek out and exercise NO! power, you won't always get what you want. But at least you'll feel better about yourself for having said or done what was good for you while respecting the rights of others: *Being assertive is more valuable than winning.*

Learning to say no can change your life. Just remember how it sounds. The next time you choose to veto an action, say any one of these:

- I must say no.
- I understand your position, but I'm afraid I can't help you.
- I can't do that. It just won't be convenient.
- No.
- No!
- NO!

# 4

## Who's Tempting the New Eve?

Della, forty-five years old now, was carefully and beautifully tailored to fit the conventional ideal of a young girl that had been established in the early 1950s—virginal, accommodating to men, just bright enough to amuse her husband-to-be, a man just starting law school. Della and Paul married when they were both twenty-one years old. She assumed Paul had had early sexual experiences, but to her surprise they were both virgins on their wedding night. She was happy to be married; sexual gratification would come later. "For a month [of marriage] I kept telling myself it was impossible to be so happy, and before you could say 'prognostication,' had the thrill of having that turn out to be absolutely true," says the heroine of *Diary of a Mad Housewife*. "In July I discovered I was pregnant, which wasn't exactly what we had in mind." Della's life paralleled that of the resigned Tina in Sue Kaufman's fictional tale. Della's next child, born a year and a half after her first, was planned.

Eight years passed; both Della's children were away from home for most of the day and Della enrolled in law school. She was twenty-nine years old. Paul did not approve of her going to school, especially in law. This was outright competition, if not treason. Her parents tried to dissuade her; his were equally disapproving of her aspirations. Paul grudgingly watched Della's ambitions materialize. Their sex life, never superb, was at a standoff.

Paul came from a household where sex was rarely discussed. And as a grown man he could not discuss it or his needs with Della. He had not been an adept lover, but an eager and vulnerable one. Now he was no lover at all. As Della sought to free herself of early restraints by seeking a career, Paul, fearing loss of control, tried to reimpose them. As a result, he behaved like many men—he worked on devaluing Della.

"By devaluing women in general," Steven Naifeh and Gregory Smith said astutely in *Why Can't Men Open Up?*, "a man can justify his own inability (disguised as unwillingness) to make himself vulnerable to a specific woman in a relationship that must be both equal and reciprocal to be truly intimate. A man may also devalue his own wife or lover specifically."

How well this described Paul during those years.

Then, at thirty, Della found Joe—a charming, muscular, easygoing construction worker she met one day at a local diner after school. She found herself seeking him out, liking his attention and flattery, but at first resisted his passes with good humor. Finally Joe won her and took her to a motel.

"I could not believe my body was feeling what I was feeling with Joe," she told me, recalling that turning point in her life. "I thought I'd never survive the evening. My responses were so strong, I thought it had to be beyond sex . . . like love, true, deep everlasting love. It had to be the kind of love a woman leaves her husband for."

Della convinced herself it *was* love. Once or twice a week she'd meet Joe at the same motel, same room. For one year she lived in a state of heightened emotions. Thoughts of Joe aroused her. Sex with Paul dwindled to nothing. Paul didn't make demands on her; she said nothing, did nothing. It was Joe, all Joe.

"I couldn't perceive it as just an affair with the man with whom, incidentally, I had my first orgasm after eight years of marriage," Della said. "It took on exceptional importance. It had to. I was raised to be a good girl—and good girls don't go out and have sex. Good girls are in love. I couldn't separate the two at all. I permitted my body to be taken and convinced myself to give my mind over, too.

"Interesting," she continued, "that no one ever asked me how Paul treated me. It was more a case of my being lucky to snag a nice guy who was going to be a lawyer. I was going to school, caring for two small children, keeping a home going. Joe was the highlight. I didn't care that he drank too much, that he was domineering, that we weren't really suited to each other. I needed to feel *something*. All the while, I couldn't forget where I came from, what I'd been taught. I was cheating on Paul, committing adultery. Now it was a matter of my being a 'bad girl' with a 'good' husband. The conflict tore me apart."

It was an extraordinary time for Della, a year when she discovered her sexuality and uncovered a few truths about her marriage to Paul. He was stable, hardworking, a nice guy, and she loved him. She wanted to stay married. It was also a time shrouded in secrecy: she couldn't talk about her affair with Joe. It had to remain confidential. Was she unusual—the sexually una-wakened married woman brought to life by a stranger?

The Kinsey Report, the first survey to chronicle the sexual behavior of Americans, tallied up what nearly 2500 women said about marital fidelity. In 1953, about 25 percent of the women interviewed reported having had extramarital affairs before the age of forty. About 6 percent of teen brides reported affairs by their twenties. Women sought outside affairs in some 9 percent of the cases, and when they reached about forty, nearly 25 percent of the respondents reported affairs. In the 1960s, Della was among the almost 35 percent of women her age who had had affairs. (Now, in the 1980s, estimates fluctuate between 45 and 50 percent.)

Romantic love endures for about two years. This was true for Della, who was forced to make a decision about Joe. "I lived with Paul," Della said. "I didn't live in that motel room once or twice a week. I could have kept that affair going forever. Joe excited me. But this fantasy world existed within a very limited time within a very limited framework." The affair took its natural course and ended.

It is often the wife's wish not to disrupt her marriage although she's having an affair. This seems paradoxical, but it can make perfect sense to the evolving New Eve, who is both a sexually experienced woman and a basically traditional wife with strong moral values. Marriage is stabilizing, effective in enough ways to satisfy her. She knows that sexual incompatibility is not a good enough reason to divorce. Had Della not wanted to live with Paul, had there been total incom-patibility on more essential levels, she'd have been wise to leave.

"I hadn't slept with Paul for nearly two years," Della

added. "I don't know what he did all that time for sexual release, and quite honestly I'm happier not knowing. Paul had failings, but he was a good husband in other ways. I wanted to make the marriage work. The first time we slept together again after I stopped seeing Joe was a shock to both of us. I came back to him as an experienced woman. Joe taught me everything. Paul made an offhand remark about my style of love-making, as in, how did I know *that?* I told him I'd been doing some reading, one of those manuals. I sensed that he didn't want to know anything further. It never went beyond that."

Della's case describes a woman who struggled to maintain a marriage and launch a career while trying to deal effectively with her newfound sexuality. The questions facing her were: Was her sexuality worth developing? How basic was it to her survival? Why did she feel so strongly inclined, after eight years of marriage and very minimal satisfaction with her husband, to seek sexual experiences? Would she just be another casualty of the sexual revolution?

Women like Della, whose sexual orientation was fixed before the era of greater openness, acceptance and freedom to explore, are beset by conflicts like these. They were expected to become sexually available to their husbands, and sexual pleasure was not mandatory according to our mothers' standards and preachings. Then the Pill freed women from fear of pregnancy, that absolute evidence of a sex life. With it came freedom to find pleasure. If you didn't, there was abundant help available from manuals, clinics and willing suitors.

Illustrated sex manuals offered vivid step-by-step directives for more fulfilling sex, and may have helped some couples. For others, sex therapy changed the nature of their intimate lives. Still others relinquished sex totally—better to just let it drift quietly away than drive it off through repeated disappointment or lack of interest. But after years of candid questing, women began to make sex a more natural and less self-conscious part of their lives, and looked for other ways to become fulfilled as human beings. They rediscovered themselves through work and a willingness to investigate the complexities of personality while struggling to keep a marriage together. So today, a New Eve is emerging from the old sexual persona. Who is she and how does the ever-present, seemingly all-important issue of sex fit into her life?

Let's go back briefly to what we all learned in the beginning. At the core of our being, we were creatures born to be sexually expressive. As children, we are all sexually demonstrative, reaching out to one another without any need to use sex to manipulate, control, or prove a point. We've been given all the equipment to experience pleasure. Even in our most innocent early days as infants, we were sexual beings—a condition our parents were not aware of or didn't quite want to accept. We had the capacity and the inclination, not yet repressed, to have unlimited and varied kinds of sexual experiences. Little boys had erections, little girls lubricated—both have orgasmic potential. As we got older, we were taught not to touch ourselves, not to touch or be touched sexually by others, not be enthralled by pleasure or give in to it.

Messages about sexuality became more explicit as we grew into adolescence. These served as inhibitory messages warning us that, in the extreme, sex was nasty, pernicious, a violation of the female body. In the milder version, but just as inhibitory in the long run, sex was exciting but taboo. As a result, forbidden sex before marriage increased in value. Stolen hours were spent together indulging in sex play—if not intercourse—with a built-in frenzied intoxication. When sex was taboo, excitement was high. We learned that excitement and sexual prohibition were a desirable erotic combination.

Warnings about sex are part of our heritage. Here are a few you've heard at the kitchen table over a number of cups of coffee with mothers, aunts, older sisters, even fathers fervently committed to keeping daughters virginal until marriage: Men are animals, gluttons out for one thing only, and you are in possession of that one thing. You must make a covenant to guard that thing with your life. Any lapse in the guardianship of your body and, you are told, you will get pregnant. Sexual abandon, then, implies instant motherhood or a befouled reputation. There is no middle ground: Have sex, get pregnant, and you will become an outcast; do not have sex and you will marry; maybe not well, but at least you will marry.

Sex came with penalties back then, not pleasure. The final warning usually sounded like this: "Have sex and you'll be sorry." And, thirty years ago, when a parent said you'd be sorry, you took it literally. There was no question that you would suffer. There was no underground system of support from friends, relatives or social organizations that would help if you were exiled from your family because you were having sex or got pregnant. The family oversaw your behavior, protected you. You did not want to be the "bad girl," the "tramp," the girl who traded her body for love or attention or whatever it was she needed from a boy.

Over yet another cup of coffee you may have been advised about the arcane business of male sexuality—most specifically, men initiate sex not only to reaffirm their ego, but to get *us* moving and responsive. Women, therefore, did not ask for sex, but waited and, when desired, responded on cue.

What was the rationale supporting this wait? Women were not supposed to be sexual beings. They had to be protected by others, especially their husbands. Sex, by this faulty reasoning, was a duty and an obligation. But what if you had sexual feelings in spite of attempts to control them? What if you wanted to initiate sex? What if you wanted to feel sexual abandon, be transported, delighted in another's arms? What if your ego wanted its own brand of protection—acceptance of your sexuality?

The Old Eve suffered these questions, and the New Eve of the 1980s faces them still. Now as before, it's a double-edged sword. Philip Blumstein and Pepper Schwartz, co-authors of the exceptional study *American Couples,* cited this conclusion: "We think husbands become more proprietary about male prerogatives when other sources of prestige and power are disturbed," they write, referring specifically to a male's feeling of vulnerability about his work or some other area of his life. ". . . Men have traditionally had the right of sexual access to their wives. This right was even written into religious and civil law, and women were expected to be sexually available as part of their duty. But if men had the right to ask for—and expect—sex, they also had the *duty* to initiate it. To this day, men take this prescription very seriously. They often become angry when they ask for sex and their partners refuse. And they also feel guilty when they do not fulfill their duty to initiate sex."

To initiate is to pursue. Men pursue, and some are brilliant practitioners of the art. Put a willing woman, who cannot let a man know the degree of her willingness, with a pursuing man, and soon she will surrender. She will submit when she feels she's convinced him that she is powerless; she has no choice—she must act out her impulses. He's pinned her down, but not brutally. He's been forceful and persistent because he knows she wants what he wants. She's governed by other laws, and he knows them by heart. She must tease, tantalize, beg him to beg her. Only then can she be lusty, because that lustiness has been brought out by a pursuer. She claims, "It's not really me. This is outside my control. He is irresistible."

Back to the kitchen table before the 1960s for another visit with the girl who *is* in control. She hears her mother or another authority figure saying that it is up to her to stop a man's advances. Men are unstoppable, goes the admonition, unless you are stronger, smarter and fleeter of foot. Eventually control becomes reflexive. For years to come it's woven into the fiber of her life. Separating sexual control from sexual pleasure, then, looms in the foreground when a girl does marry. Her wedding night blesses her surrender. So the Old Eve placed her first priority on getting married. It established her as a normal, conventional woman who would give over the greater part of her life to husband and family, keeping a home.

But even then she remained controlled. If she lost control—showed how she enjoyed sex—she would be giving her body over to the enemy. The fable says he would abuse her, misuse her, attempt to have intercourse with her at his whim and fancy. She would be his puppet.

For many of us, the thrill was not in connubial pleasures, but in the fact that "he wanted us"—he married us. For the Old Eve, the only control she could count on was control over her body—her last reserve of power. If she gave that up, she lost herself completely. She no longer existed except for him. Sex was an interaction of loving bodies pleasing each other, but not for her. For her, sex was something done to take care of her husband, tolerating his fondling. The Old Eve was less likely to "make love" in those days; she "had sex." And sex brought her, if nothing else, a man's affiliation and fidelity. Sex was her greatest performance. She was what she was taught to be—a sexual actress. This was once the basis of countless marriages.

And so the Old Eve controlled a man by denial when she could. As she refused him access to her body, so the battles increased. Her husband called her "frigid"—a word we don't hear much lately. Physiology often helped her out—she tightened up, not permitting penetration. And, then, all those decades back, the controlled Eve may have opted to deny herself pleasure by not allowing her husband to know he could please her. In many ways the only power she may have had was over her own body. If she had to deny herself pleasure to prove that power, then she did.

The Old Eve got older, just old enough to be in her prime—her late twenties or early thirties, perhaps with a child or two—when the sexual revolution fired some shocking new cannons in her direction. Now it was okay to be sexual! Most men were conflicted over the new rules. They appreciated a woman's sudden availability but still hesitated to accept her sexuality full force. We all know men who took sides during the revolution ("Bring back the virgins" versus "Bring on the girls"). Women took sides too, and many of them wound up being their own worst enemies—"I've given, but what have I gotten?"

At one time, being a pleaser in bed for a man's sake elevated a woman to the status of good sexual partner;

now she could be a "good" sexual partner by being pleased *by* him. But how was she to be pleased? Freud made the pronouncement that the vaginal orgasm was the only acceptable indication of a woman's true femininity. The clitoral orgasm characterized her as "masculine." So, after centuries of denying women any sort of sexuality, we now had to locate the orgasm somewhere or other on our bodies and make incorrect judgments on where it did or did not originate. This situation remained until sex researchers Masters and Johnson cleared up the information and proved that all orgasms involve the clitoris whether or not there is direct stimulation.

Confused? Many women were. Some gave a momentary shudder when the social norms changed from traditional restraint to a new ideology that bestowed upon them the *right* to sexual exploration, and, not caring, stayed as they were. Others gave up sexual suppression and took lovers by the dozen. However, multiple experiences did not guarantee pleasure, healthy relationships with men, or self-esteem. They may just have guaranteed dates! Maybe the Old Eve had a point, many disillusioned women opined. Restraint at least didn't hurt or reject you.

## The New Eve

Those of us who have come through these decades sane, functioning and fairly happy as sexual and compassionate human beings quite simply deserve tributes, applause, a medal! We have survived the myths and claims about female sexuality and the shifting ideologies that wanted to authorize how we should feel and where we should feel it. Some of us have had enough courage to discover our sexuality and know what pleases us. It may be sexual involvement with one man or with many men; no sex, some sex, or a lot of sex; bisexuality; homosexuality; extramarital sex. We are the New Eves, the transitional generation. Our mothers, most of them, are probably still locked into the old rules of submitting by obligation—where any sexual response is a bonus. The 1980s teenager, having grown up with omnipresent sexual stimulation, is indulging in sexual behavior at an earlier age, but not necessarily enjoying it or understanding its impact any better than we did when we started on our journeys.

The New Eve is a smart cookie and she celebrates her new sexual maturity in a variety of ways. Let's look at some of them.

# Separating Love and Sex

The New Eve can meet the challenge of separating love and sex when they must be separated, and joining them again when it's in her best interest to do so. Often a woman can feel deprived, undesirable, hungry for attention. A man catches her eye. He wants her. She wants him, needs his affirmation. What's happening? Not necessarily the basis for love, but a powerful chemical connection between two people. Swept away by romantic dreams, she places him in an exalted position. Her desire transforms his responses into profound meaning. "He sees me as *me*," the Old Eve would have declared, insisting that the sexual response be made into something grander, worthier. "He brings out the best in me . . . I've never felt this way before . . . What we have is different!"

Every woman has felt this way at least once. Her

desire is so great that she believes she'll die if she never touches the man again. Encounters with him are heated. She cannot imagine any man ever affecting her again. This is sex. Good sex.

I do not suggest that you excise such a heady experience from your life. I do beseech you to know its place in the scheme of things. If it is sex that keeps you with a man, acknowledge it, as Della did. You are not obliged to love this man because he's the right lover for you, nor should you confuse his sexual attraction to you as an indication of eventual commitment. My appeal to women caught up in torrid encounters is to defuse the power of sex by having a sense of humor about what happens between you. I don't mean that you should mock yourself, but free yourself. Relish the sex, enjoy it the way you'd enjoy a blissfully content day at the beach. If it is sex that enthralls you, figure out what it is about the man that does it for you. Is it truly his style? Is he seductive, excessively flattering and attentive? Does he convince you that you are the only woman in the world who moves *him*? But what about those flash fights that happen all the time when you're together—except when you are in each other's arms? Do doubt, confusion or anger excite both of you? Is he really giving, or giving you a hard time?

The New Eve, I hope, will evaluate what sex means to her and make choices that will not hurt her in the long run. If an experience is essentially sexual, the New Eve can know when to begin a relationship and when to end it. Who is the man? What's really wanted here? Desire is not enough. The New Eve has the courage to say to the interested man, "I really like you, but no, I can't see you. Perhaps under other circumstances, another time, it might have been terrific." Endings are tougher. The New Eve must be strong enough to face the breakup of an exclusively sexual relationship with, "It was wonderful, but now it's over." The New Eve knows that every good lover isn't necessarily a good person to love.

# Sex Is Ever-Changing

Sex is not orderly, consistent or predictable. The New Eve accepts elements of change in sexual desire from high to low and low to high. These shifts can be temporary or they can establish long-term trends. Our attitudes about sex are altered depending on circumstances and the varied pressures we experience. These influence how much or how little sex we want. As we get older, our tastes and proclivities may swing one way or another, reverse themselves or successfully remain the same. Novelty may amuse us or a new sexuality may be distilled to utmost clarity from a formerly cloudy brew.

The form sexual activity takes is not immutable. The New Eve need not look any further than herself in searching for a reason why her tastes have changed. They just have. At the heart of the matter is personal growth or a changing of roles.

Sexual expression may shift, for example, while a woman is pregnant or after having a child. In *Sexual Turning Points*, Lorna J. Sarrel and Philip M. Sarrel, MD, cite a number of studies that describe what happens during these exceptional stages. The authors stress that heightened or lessened sexual interest during pregnancy is largely a matter of "individual variation." There is no "correct" way to behave. During the first trimester, many women may have a weaker libido because they're worried about hurting the fetus, and some suffer from fatigue or nausea. Others experience no change. During the second trimester, a woman may not only experience heightened sexuality but "may have the most intense orgasms she has ever experienced. Some women who are not ordinarily multiorgasmic have multiple orgasms." The reason the authors cite is more physiological than psychological. Others, they found, were "completely turned off" at this stage.

In the last trimester, the Sarrels write, "all studies agree that sexual activity declines in the seventh, eighth and ninth months of pregnancy, and most sharply of all in the ninth month. Discomfort during intercourse is one commonly given reason for decline in intercourse toward the end of pregnancy." Finally, the study found that "new parents are likely to show a decline in intercourse frequency throughout the first year after their baby's birth."

Sex is ever-changing not only for the New Eve, but also for the New Adam, who may still be bristling with holdover attitudes from his life as the Old Adam. Liberation is not always equitable. After having a new child, some women become centered on the baby and are not as attentive to a husband's needs. Conflict may arise within him about having sex with a "mother," even though that mother is also his wife, the woman he loves and desired before the child was born.

What's the solution? This will take patience and diplomacy—for both of you. During your child's first year, it may be tempting to let the sexual relationship decline. Caring for a newborn is a formidable task. But it is within the New Eve's power to encourage her husband to relate to her as a sexual partner as well as the mother of his children. This is a wonderful opportunity for you to practice a bit of sexual assertion that's really quite simple and time-tested in its effectiveness. Prepare a romantic evening. First hire a babysitter and then check into a motel for a few hours. This is the evening to become sexually reacquainted, the evening you can affirm your husband's desirability and present yourself as a woman who is both a nurturing mother and an attentive, lusty woman.

# Some Women Prefer Women

The New Eve may confront formerly forbidden tendencies and declare that she prefers her sexual partners to be women, not men. Denial no longer seems necessary. In actual practice, it is acculturation, religious adherence, and discomfort with homosexuality that prevent a great proportion of us from expressing our preferences.

During the mid-1970s, many women reached out sexually to other women while embracing "sisterhood." Whether or not long-lasting relationships developed from these forays into homosexuality was not the point. Sometimes these sexual encounters were just experimentation. They answered the question, What's it like to be with a person who shares the same anatomy, a similar emotional and social history? For others, motives were more a result of trendiness than attachment—it was suddenly okay to be with a woman and to march for the right to do so. A number of women found love and solace. I once spoke to a woman of nineteen who had had two unhappy relationships with men. Self-esteem was low; she felt unloved, especially unattractive, in turmoil. She met an older woman and got caught up in her attentions, finding the love and care so missing from her life. Tina was convinced she was gay. A year later she was dating men again. Was she "homosexual"? For Tina, it was a sexual interlude with depth, caring, and mutual physical pleasure. Homosexuality was secondary now, and did not determine the course of her life. The affair was a valuable experience for her.

Tina thought that no man could want her, that it would take a woman to care. She interpreted her connection to a woman as an irreversible choice about her sexuality. She was gay, that was it. But she wasn't. It was more awareness that her sexuality could change, depending on life's conditions, that permitted her to move to another level of behavior.

When the New Eve ventures into an entirely different sexual arena, she can view it as transitional or long term. She can discriminate between the levels of her sexuality and know that this is who she is *now*, this is how she feels *now*, but she's not sure how long she'll feel this way.

In a number of Mediterranean and Arab cultures it's perfectly acceptable for grown-up heterosexual men to hold hands or embrace in public and not be branded as gay. Not in America. In America, men shake hands, clap shoulders like good buddies, hug each other for triumphs, but they don't do anything as romantically symbolic as holding hands. But heterosexual women have always embraced each other, held hands, stroked each other in a friendly fashion, fussed over each other's hair and seen each other bare as babes. And it is accounted as little more than comfort at being with each other, tenderness, a fine intimacy that's cherished. If there are sexual overtones, they are often suppressed or unexpressed. Moments of extreme intimacy may or may not translate into sexual tension. Women can hug and hold each other and settle for that.

There are women, too, who've suddenly made a choice that belies the rest of their lives. After a lifetime of heterosexuality, they meet a woman who matters to them beyond friendship. Celia, at forty-nine, after four children and twenty-four years of marriage to the only man she'd ever slept with, found Georgia, a thirty-seven-year-old antiques dealer and "fell in love no matter how hard I tried not to."

Celia carried on an emotionally and physically stimulating affair without her husband's knowledge. He found them together one day. Tom was intolerably shocked, yet he wanted to remain married to Celia. He demanded she give up her lover. Celia wanted marriage *and* Georgia. Celia's resolution was too painful for Tom to handle; she was forced to leave.

Now Celia faced an interesting dilemma. She's not adjusted enough to be publicly gay, though Georgia is happy to be who she is quite openly. Celia loves Georgia and has finally agreed to live with her. To do so comfortably, they've had to relocate. In a new environment Celia will be able to fully test her commitment to Georgia. Here she can define her homosexuality or discover if she's just going through a phase. If she's gay, she's gay. If she's not, she will have to go on and build a different life.

Blumstein and Schwartz place homosexual women in historical perspective in *American Couples*. From earliest times, female friendships have been encouraged, and close relationships between women have been permitted because they were not imagined to be sexual. "Women were allowed a latitude of emotional expression so they could use words reserved for lovers and not be aware that their affection and commitment could also be sexual." They wrote impassioned notes to each other, declared their love, lived together, traveled as friends. But when women took on male trappings—tailored suits, cropped hair, masculine gestures—they were censured. "She" walked as fine an edge as "he."

For most of history, close female relationships were thought to be, *au fond*, innocent, because women were not given credit for sexuality. According to Schwartz and Blumstein, even if close friendships were suspected of being physically intimate, they were not seen as a "threat to the established order since no illegitimate heir could result from a woman's relationship with another woman." This was truly a man's world. Sexual legitimacy did not coexist with birthright.

Schwartz and Blumstein noted, too, a conclusion drawn by author Lillian Faderman: "Romantic friendships between young women in previous centuries were often encouraged as 'training' for heterosexual marriage. Sensitivities could be developed so that women's gentler nature would blossom even more and be of great benefit to their future husbands."

Freud thought sexuality was a normal expression of the human condition, while homosexuality showed the person to be "stuck" in the homosexual phase, a phase everyone goes through in youth. Ergo, they were not "sick" individuals but "regressed" individuals.

Studies abound, but we still do not know what combination of factors produces a homosexual. I've met men who swore they were aware of being gay at eight years old. I've met women who argued the same conclusion—their early years determined their sexuality and they never swerved from this sexual potential. There is probably a formula somewhere that records a measure of biochemical vulnerability, a confused sense of identity in conjunction with upbringing, and certain cultural cues that create the homosexual. Sex researcher Alfred Kinsey, who had no answer either, devised a rating scale graduated from 0 to 6, with total heterosexuality at one end and total homosexuality at the opposite. In the 1950s, he found that about 13 percent of the male population was predominantly gay, and about 20 percent of the male population had homosexual tendencies. The percentages for women at the time were lower for both categories, but demonstrated that a good number of women did desire other women. I don't know if there are more homosexuals now than when Kinsey made his charts, or if there is more openness in expressing these impulses.

If homosexuality becomes an unexpected revelation for you, know who you are and what this means to you. Do not concern yourself with labels, but rather focus on your needs. It's your experiential self that will dictate how you behave. Your sexuality is yours to express as long as it's not irresponsible, indiscriminate or exploited by someone else. You have the freedom to make your choice. Others may clobber you with arguments to remain one way or the other. Heterosexuals may plead with you to remain heterosexual and homosexuals may press you to be homosexual. Try to resist both groups. It's up to you alone. When you decide *your* way, there's not only comfort inherent in your choice, but it also shows an ability to be in touch with your sexuality at any particular time.

# Sexual Development Has Many Levels

The New Eve deals with the natural bent of her sexual inclinations. With all the exposure to sexual and erotic literature, X-rated films, and tales of sexual exploits bandied about by female friends, she may worry if she is just not interested in sex. But, for the New Eve, the sexual adventure is hers to choose or to not choose. If she's never had much pleasure during sex and does not try to find it, then so be it. Well-meaning friends may offer plentiful advice on how to develop her sexuality—with lovers, masturbation, gadgets, group sex, whatever—but for her, instruction manuals may be about as fascinating and as useful as a text on soil mechanics—they don't work. Or she finds that it's like reading a book on how to swim—information and experience are not the same; there's a chance she might sink.

It may not be in this Eve's best interest to develop her sexuality. She can't handle "playing with fire." What if she's suddenly a sexual being, she thinks warily, and her husband is not? Or what if he's not an adequate lover for her? What if she goes through a phase of needing lovers outside marriage? What if she experiments with sexuality and it turns out she doesn't need very much sex in order to be happy—just as she had thought at the start?

Life doesn't depend on developing intense sexuality. It is one satisfying part of life, but not all of life. How the New Eve deals with her sexuality is no one's business but her own.

## Should She or Shouldn't She?

The New Eve is grown up enough to establish her own sexual values, not wait for others to dictate them to her. Single and divorced women still face the dilemma of first, second and third date sexual etiquette. The goodnight kiss of the 1950s has become a more serious sexual wrap-up to an evening in the 1970s and 1980s, and it's troubling us. Sexual intimacy with a virtual stranger may not be the rule, but some women feel an increasing pressure to seduce or succumb far sooner than is comfortable for them. "If I don't go to bed with him," goes the familiar cry, "someone else *will* and he'll stop seeing me!"

If you suffer from "morning after" depression, hugging your knees and wondering why you agreed to sexual intimacy, know a few things: The man will stop seeing you, if that's his intention, whether or not you went to bed with him. Naturally there are other outcomes. He may call, persist, and it could be you who ends the relationship. Or, when you two finally click, there's the chance of it leading to a long-term relationship or marriage. But . . . trading sex for the possibility of love, or having sex with a man just to get there before another woman claims him, does little for your self-esteem. If sudden sex makes you suffer, refuse it.

I believe there are many men who feel pressured to attempt sexual intimacy after a short acquaintanceship with a woman. It may not be desire that motivates them, but a misguided sense of obligation to fulfill some sort of strategic expectation—that is, dinner, dessert, bed. He knows she is a woman with some sexual experience, and he is a man with sexual experience. Therefore, he reasons, she must be waiting for the inevitable. Some men are wise enough to end the evening when it should end for them. They have fears, as do women, that their bodies aren't in the greatest shape, or they may have performance problems with a woman they do not know well. They need familiarity and caring before allowing themselves to be sexually vulnerable. This man is happy to know a woman, but it is unnecessary for him to know her any better on this particular evening. Other men may be perfectly capable of fast sexual encounters—hit-and-run lovers who see no reason *not* to try, or insecure men who require intimacy as proof of their potency.

If a man enjoys you, he will see you again. Ask a man about his great love, and he will conjure up images of her even if he hasn't seen her for the greater part of his lifetime. He will describe moments of intense connection, humorous anecdotes about her eccentricities, the good feelings he had with her—most likely he won't tell you he fell for her because she was great in bed.

Some women tell me that they've given in on a first, second, or third date merely to quench a sexual craving. The man, quite honestly, could have been any male who did not have a communicable disease or a prison record. He was there at the right time. Something happened to these women, though: that empty, dreaded sensation the next day. Was it truly a sexual encounter they needed? Or did they hope for an emotional connection? If they had wanted to get laid, to be blunt, they needn't have confused sex with love. The experience is spelled L-A-I-D, not L-O-V-E.

I want to remind women that in this age ahead of us it will be crucial to behave in a fashion that's comfortable for *them*, not necessarily what's comfort-producing for someone else. There's a tremendous sense of integrity and power gained in knowing you've made the choice that matters to you. Remember, when a man penetrates your body, he penetrates your mind.

Put in perspective, sex is a fulfilling, exciting aspect of a woman's life. It is friendship first—a trusting and communicative relationship that produces warmth, affection and pleasure. Volcanic sex, ecstatic sex do not last. The New Eve does not marry for the bed only; she marries out of healthy compatibility.

It's my belief that the greatest potential for sexual growth can occur within marriage when a couple is united in the decision to make it so. Marriage is often the only place where a woman feels safe enough to shed inhibitions. She feels good about herself; her femininity and desirability can be affirmed with the marriage. She can afford to ask for what she wants from someone who cares for her. She can reveal herself in a secure setting where sexual development can be encouraged. It's a chance to act out fantasies and maintain the aura of courtship without overinflated expectations.

The New Eve has real opportunities open to her in sexual relationships. They will be conducted overwhelmingly on her terms, depending on what she is willing to become and allow to happen.

# 5

---

# From I Do to I Don't and Back to I Do

Bob, playing Sunday gardener, shirtless and baking in the heavy July heat, is singing along with a sixties rock hit that thunders from a neighbor's transistor. Kneeling now, he pokes around in a circular flower bed, replacing decapitated seedlings; the dog stalks a gardening glove. It's a friendly, familiar setting, seemingly without conflict—until his wife, Martha, arrives on the scene.

Martha catches sight of Bob from her vantage point at the living room window. She loves Bob and she loves the garden, but put one with the other and all logic is swept deliriously to one side. She feels a mixture of anger and hurt flash like lightning before her eyes. After seventeen years of marriage, Bob's triumphs of ineptitude in the backyard have gotten to her once again.

Bob is unaware of Martha or her fury—he's adrift in his own unpoetic but well-meaning fantasy about these few square yards of land behind their small suburban house. His approach to backyard work has been the same for seventeen years: he applies simple economics and simple logic and winds up with—do it yourself and

152

save money. Getting it done, not beauty or expertise, counts.

Martha would agree that the backyard looks trimmed, but it isn't what she envisioned for her garden—colorful border plants, a vegetable patch, rows of dahlias, a few exotic blooms, pruned not bandaged maples, a lawn mowed by an expert gifted on the tractor.

Bob and Martha have not spoken in five years about hiring help for the backyard. For ten years before that, the issue of the yard sparked intense battles about money, or, more accurately, the spending of money on "unnecessary obligations." Spending is painful for Bob. Though Martha works and brings home nearly as much money as her husband, he hasn't allowed her to pay for help either, believing that he somehow would end up with the entire bill anyway.

Now, as she watches Bob under the hot, dazzling sky Martha has a thought that suddenly calms her. She will go ahead with her plan. Three days later, she hires someone to clear up and plant the backyard while Bob's at work. She pays for the landscaping and intends to keep the cost from her husband; the work will take about four days.

What will happen when Bob notices the backyard in progress? Martha worries. Another blow-up perhaps, accusations that she's extravagant and shows disregard and disrespect for how hard he works . . . Martha decides not to torture herself with premature visions of Bob's displeasure. Bob returns home later; Martha takes him to the back door to view the bone of contention. She assures him he'll like the results and that the pleasure of his own miniature park won't cost him a cent. Bob is distrustful but lets it ride. This is not like him—momentarily, Martha fears for her marriage. Finally, the landscaping is done. Bob loves it!

Keeping her agreement with herself, Martha doesn't mention or intimate the cost of the job, and Bob doesn't ask. He loves the backyard; though pleased with her decision, Martha experiences mixed feelings.

All those years she feared Bob's reaction to her going ahead and changing the rules by changing the status quo. This was risky. "Would he leave me or torment me with the details of how I'd ruined everything by acting without consulting him?" Martha worried. "Those fears kept me quietly seething."

Then she had a revelation, a shockingly simple revelation—Bob is Bob and no argument she might present would change him. "If this had only occurred to me ten years before!" she said. "Bob is limited when it comes to money; and that's it. I did not want it to limit *me* any longer. I took a big chance, I know I did, and it's *freed* me.

"But let me tell you what pains me about this experience," Martha says with a catch in her voice. "For as long as we've had this house, the yard and what to do about it was a recurring issue. Did we really need to argue so bitterly about it? Did he really have to make me feel that I was a fool with money, both his and mine, for wanting a nicer backyard than he had in mind? Can you understand that while I'm happy Bob likes what I've done, I'm still a bit resentful for his having begrudged me what, it turns out, *both* of us enjoy."

Martha's story fascinated me on so many levels. First and most obviously, Martha could easily represent any woman who's had a love relationship with a man, within or without marriage. She could be any woman who has, on occasion, almost *defined* the relationship by the problem most likely to recur and remain unresolved within it. In Martha's case, the issue of spending and not spending persisted. The marriage, then, was "about" their views on money rather than, for example, struggles such as "his mother," "her father," how a child is raised, infidelity, drinking, his domination, her controlling behavior, his temper, her health. Each relationship takes its own form depending upon the personalities influencing it.

Martha's is an interesting story. She went from "I do" to "I don't" and back to "I do" again. How did this happen?

Any woman who's been married can tell me her own version of "the backyard"—and perhaps the resolution wasn't as pleasant as in Martha's case. After all, Martha got what she wanted by taking the initiative. This satisfied her, and, eventually, Bob. As you might imagine, not every husband would be as agreeable as Bob upon discovering his backyard under construction, especially without his consent or participation. But many husbands *can* be as agreeable as Bob, though it may seem unbelievable to you now. The point is that a daring action is what set Martha apart from so many married women who go through lifetimes of frustration, never taking the step that can *change the marriage, not the man.*

If there is one thing I want to stress in these pages it's this thought: *Change your expectations within the relationship, and you can change your life!* If your marriage has evolved from the joyous and hopeful state of "I do" to the divisive and confusing state of "I don't," there is still a chance for you to retrieve some of that original joy that brought you two together and get back to "I do."

Let's backtrack a moment to Martha. Like many women, she was conditioned to be a pleaser. Her purpose in the marriage was to create comfort for Bob—emotional and physical comfort. She believed this was right. Bob functioned as the dutiful husband, providing security and steadfastness. He regarded his role as right, too. Over the years, each learned the other's limitations, shortcomings and strengths. Each was poignantly aware of what caused anguish, happiness, anger, tenderness, sexual tension or significant fears of abandonment in the other. Martha would say she knew Bob as no other could; Bob would say he understood what made Martha Martha.

Yet, for seventeen years Martha argued and fought for control with Bob over money. Hundreds of spats or full-blown bitter disputes later, Martha had not converted Bob from a seriously frugal to an even marginally fair spender. He was overinvolved with money and its meaning for him; she was overinvolved in challenging Bob's fervent commitment to *not* spending. If you're always being challenged on some point in your character, would you change it in a flash just because someone demanded it? Most men won't.

So here's Martha before the miracle of having the backyard done to her satisfaction—a woman determined to convert Bob so he'd open the purse strings, at least to let in some light. She's had practice—nearly twenty years of it. Of course Bob has said yes to some purchases—smaller ones or those he wanted for himself. In those cases, Martha got her bouquet of roses, so to speak, when her husband agreed to pay for or share the expense for something she wanted. When requests were vetoed, what happened then?

A "no" usually launched an attempt by Martha to triumph in an impossible task—changing Bob's mind.

Women set out to convert men in different ways. Some complain loudly for years, or are angry, withdrawn and silent when the thorny subject arises. The result: a husband may submit or not. Other women cry, threaten or resort to trickery. Again, the result is that he may or may not give in. Martha, being a reasonable enough woman, began by presenting Bob with a nice, sane case for what she wanted. Bob, a nice, sane man, listened attentively and said no. Martha became irritated, braced herself, then raised her voice. Bob responded in a louder voice. Then Martha and Bob tested each other, verbally pushed each other and got nowhere. Here we are now, seventeen years later.

What changed Martha? Did Bob change without Martha's knowing it? Did Bob set things up so Martha would pay? She tells it this way:

"In order for me to love Bob and live with him for the remainder of our lives," Martha said with feeling, "I have to accept him as the person he is. How simple that is to say, but it's taken me this long to say it, take it in . . . to believe it in my heart.

"I'm not going to make a hero out of a nice guy, and Bob's just a nice guy—a man who doesn't like to spend money, take many risks or experience life with a sense of adventure. For all those years I didn't accept Bob as he is and got myself into trouble. I spent all that time worrying about what he'd do *if*. I knew Bob all along, though, and didn't know I knew him! He was a man who wouldn't mind if things were taken care of and didn't have to know what they cost if he wasn't writing the checks. He argued out of some false pride, but truly didn't care if *I* paid for what I wanted. In its way, that little plot of backyard changed my marriage."

Martha has brought up a number of points that are important for you to examine with respect to your own marriage if it has gone from "I do" to "I don't." I'll pose them as questions for you.

• Are you accepting your husband as he is?
• Do you live on contingencies, not acting because you fear what your husband will do *if?*
• Do you know your husband, but pretend you do not by always reacting with surprise to his responses?
• Or, do you know your husband but continue to hold on to the hope that tomorrow he will miraculously change?

The answers to these questions may be complicated, but they will show if you can *love and let be.* If you can love and let be, taking the next step to change the marriage and not the man will be a lot easier. Martha discovered a simple conclusion and you can, too: This is who my husband is and either I'm going to be married to who he is or not. If he is going to change, it must be of his own free will. Bob will never have immense curiosity or a sense of adventure and certainly not a philanthropic nature; Martha knows this. Accepting Bob as singularly Bob relieved the enormous tension in her marriage. She was able to give up the dream of his being transformed into a husband who was more giving—emotionally, socially and financially. "Sometimes I think he could give me more," Martha commented, "but he's just not going to. Now that's okay, but I had to make peace with it."

When we compare a husband to a fantasy that we've created about him and he doesn't come through by actualizing it, we tamper with and often destroy our ability to enjoy the man for who he is. Instead, we accuse him of each way that he has failed to live up to our image of him. We want him to be an adult, to be a success, to be more passionate, to take care of us in splendid ways. For example: If you are married to a small-town car salesman but you fancy yourself in a glamorous marriage, wedded to a dashing and successful corporate head in the auto business like Lee Iacocca, you would do better to find the man who is as ambitious for himself as you are for him. Compare your car salesman to Lee Iacocca and you won't have much of a marriage. You'll have a husband who's bitter over not achieving the goals you've set for him and who feels profound disappointment in not being the person you wanted him to be.

If you hold every one of those disappointments against him (he's cheap, he's not sexy enough, he's insensitive, he tries to take over my life on every level, and so on), the marriage will go from "I do" to "I don't" pretty quickly.

Since many of our difficulties originate with our feelings about marriage, let's look at why we *do* marry, then examine the steps that take us from "I do" to "I don't."

# What Do We Think About Marriage?

I came across some fascinating statistics about marriage. We are still a traditional nation—90 percent of all Americans expect to marry. The percentage of us who choose spouses from groups outside our own has increased enormously—interracial marriages have more than doubled since 1970, and 21 percent of women marry younger men. If the marriage doesn't work out, singlehood of one or both ex-spouses doesn't last long—seven out of ten divorced people decide to remarry within five years of the divorce. And just a quick figure on divorce: it's more than quadrupled since 1960, with the average marriage lasting 6.8 years. While only 68.8 percent of formerly married women remarry, their ex-spouses go to the altar again at the rate of 78.3 percent. (Married men are the happiest subgroup in America, remember, and they clearly expect to keep it that way.)

We're marrying, we shall always marry, and we shall always find marriage problematic, but also alluring and comforting nevertheless. Marriage is the deepest form of connection between two people. Intimacy, true intimacy, is bliss. But we are human—bliss is not a consistent state of mind. Our differences do turn up, and then life isn't quite so blissful when issues become powder kegs. And guess what? We blame *marriage*—marriage as a thing apart from us, as if it were something that could come alive and be nice to us, not a unique interaction between two people.

So marriage got a bad name years back. The news of its fall from grace was shocking—much like the disclosure that a clergyman is corrupt. And so we must ask: Dare we commit ourselves to this institution or will we be made fools of?

A short while back, singlehood was de rigueur. Designers turned their talents to streamlining apartments, appurtenances, and appearances for the unmarried. The family circle was shrinking, and colonies of singles congregated, often becoming improvised families.

As it happened, singlehood was not a replacement for marriage. Women still felt an overwhelming wish for "oneness," both in and out of marriage. As a single person, some felt disconnected, isolated, displaced. So marriage became fashionable again—but it wasn't the same. Women had tasted the joys of independence and individuality and didn't want to give them up. They feared that in marriage, the two of you were to be "one," and the one typically took on the husband's philosophies and personality. "Looking for independence," says Megan Marshall in *The Cost of Loving,* women most often found isolation as they stopped creating families and began creating careers. "To say you didn't love your job," she says astutely, "was like our mothers saying they didn't love their husbands. It was an admission of failure."

Something interesting happened when the single style was "in." Without a *balance* between love and work, many women developed a fear of intimacy as they involved themselves more in the outside workings of the world and less with emotional fulfillment through a family. Marshall offers an analysis of this phenomenon: "While men instinctively knew fears of intimacy would pass, many women . . . adopted it as a way of life. And when men eventually decided to marry, they never had to ask themselves whether they were setting a bad example for mankind, or whether they were compromising the struggle for man's independence. Women tormented themselves endlessly with such questions."

Within marriage, women who sought self-expression may have confronted husbands who did not approve of such unwifely endeavors. These women sought a balance, but for a number of personal reasons, work—work that mattered to them—appeared out of reach. I know, it's the 1980s. People ask in surprise, Do women *still* fret over whether or not to get a job? It's so common, so accepted—what's the problem? Do men *still* exert such a limiting force over women? Or is it women themselves who set up arbitrary boundaries and change them as goals get nearer and nearer? Do women set up situations so they fail? How do we go from "I do" to "I don't"?

Not surprisingly, one reason can be, among others, the magic of romance. Here's how that works.

# Romance: Too Much of a Good Thing

Life between the two of you isn't as neat as it was that first year of marriage—the year you were still a little breathless with passion for your husband, when plans seemed so vivid, positive and *possible*. Years and years later, your beloved now belies the dream. Your prince is a pauper; your high school football hero never made the pros and now sells shoes in a shopping center; the charming boy you fell for now distributes his favors to any women who'll say yes; the sensitive, high-strung man you married provokes arguments or finds fault with you so he can express himself violently.

Think of those early days, though, and you can be psychologically aroused again. They were wonderful. You both agreed on how your world would work and you put so much effort into perpetuating the motion that kept it working. Time passed. A lot of time. It's the 1980s. You and your husband no longer agree on how the world works—in fact, you dream of other worlds where you can escape from unjustified emotional or financial deprivation. You are *frustrated*. You yearn for breathless passion once more.

Author Carol Cassell described it so well in her book *Swept Away:* "Again and again, I've been taken aback by the lack of connection between a woman's love fantasy and the world's reality." How persistently true this is for some women! Not long ago, a forty-two-year-old woman who's a perfect example of it came to see me. The problem was that Diana's husband, upon approaching fifty, intended to fulfill a secret dream—to act out all his as yet unexpressed sexual fantasies, with Diana as star participant. She agreed to some kinky scenarios, but she knew it would have to end. By the time these sexual plays began, the marriage had been faltering for five years as George seized more and more power that kept Diana trapped within his old promises to "take care of her."

Diana wanted to leave her husband. She was convinced he didn't love her; she doubted her love for him. But she needed George, needed his financial support for herself and her three sons. One day Diana met Frank, a twenty-six-year-old superannuated hippie who worked part time in a bookshop and part time as a waiter and composed blues songs, "his true calling." Despite her better judgment, she began spending two afternoons a week at his apartment.

One morning, Diana came to see me—joyous, incandescent, full of news. Yes, she'd decided to leave George and go off with Frank to Santa Fe. Was I happy for her? She'd actually made a decision. In fact, two of them—she'd leave George and join Frank.

What does it mean, this running off together? What was she thinking when she agreed to this plan? "We love each other," Diana says. What will she do about her two younger sons—especially since one has a disability? Will they go with her? Diana answers vaguely:

163

"Maybe. We haven't quite figured that one out." Where will you live? Diana: "Frank hasn't found an apartment yet, but he will." What will Frank do in Santa Fe? Diana: "Get a job." Doing what? I ask. "It doesn't matter," Diana tells me. "He'll find one." What, exactly, does Frank have? What does he hold for her? "He's young, he's sexy, he's poetic, he makes me feel desirable," Diana says, then adds, "he makes me feel like I'm worth something."

Diana feels her marriage is a dreadful failure and Frank's offer seemed to restore faith in her ability to make connections, create love, dream about a future. But this is certainly not clarity of vision. This is not self-protection. This has nothing to do with heeding the clues that can tip you off to imminent self-destructive behavior. Diana's decision came from high levels of adrenaline and other laboratory-scrutinized chemicals our brains and organs secrete upon arousal. Her plan to leave George for Frank is caused by the phenomenon of *romance*—a releaser of fantasies accompanied by some exceptionally arousing chemical reactions.

What is Diana really doing? She is leaping from a relationship with an overbearing, emotionally stunted husband who has not worked through his sexual problems to an unfocused sexual dreamer who will improvise a living with or without her. What's really going on here?

Diana's first error is in using Frank as an emergency exit out of her relationship with George. This time, she thinks, life will be different. Why? She's being guided by heady notions of a perfect relationship based on romantic inclinations. But founding a relationship on romance does not assure success with a man the next time around—for Diana or for any woman.

Since Frank does not behave the way George does, Diana falsely assumes that she's chosen a man who's better for her. The truth tells another story: not all of us learn from our mistakes. Therefore, the problems we have in relating to a "George" will be duplicated in how we relate to a more idealized "Frank." *Unless we examine the dynamics behind our problems, we will basically replicate the conditions of an unsatisfactory relationship with a man over and over again.* So George may be an overbearing husband to Diana, but there has also been some cooperation on Diana's part—she needs him, in some way, to structure her life according to his wishes. Frank, a nice guy, may be more laid back in style, but he's still got power over her—she's ready to live his life, *his* way. Frank supplied the patina of romance and Diana was fooled.

Diana's second error stems from a confusion common among romantics: she believes that a good lover is a good man to love. The reverse may often be closer to the truth: *A good lover is not necessarily a good man to love.* Since she's romantic, she's using that romanticism to confirm her desirability as a woman of forty-two, and to help disconnect her from the brutally real situation of a possibly lost marriage. Diana feels wanted, successful as a woman, because Frank is younger, a free spirit, someone new and affirming in her life. She is her own favorite heroine right now; Frank encourages the confectionary image.

Diana is real, though, and fictionalized heroines are not. Heroines who live on the page dazzle us in torrid, sweeping sagas. Headstrong but lovable women, they are fully outfitted with quicksilver temperaments, jewel-like eyes, pearly skin, tapering waists and a charm that's irresistible to any man they encounter—

but especially to the hero. The fictional hero (unlike Frank) will be prosperous and unattainable; like Frank he will seem to stand tall and defy convention as he quirks his heavy, expressive brows, exasperating the heroine and offering cruel, sardonic grins before, at last, that first melting kiss. The hero is an interesting man with a mission. The heroine is beautiful but flawed and the hero pursues her across continents and over spans of years until, finally, they confess their innermost thoughts and deep, abiding love for each other. A $400-million-a-year business in romance novels testifies to how millions of women yearn for such tales. How tantalizing it sounds, as I describe it, and how totally unreal it is. Like many women, Diana has built a fantasy and wants to live in it. She thinks "life" will take care of her; love will never falter and certainly not perish. These are possibilities the romance novel heroine totally supports—the happy ending. Diana could not have predicted, in her early forties, that a man such as Frank could have made a difference.

There are many women who understand Diana's plight—the need to replace one man with his idealized version, even if the search for the ideal becomes a way of life, a perpetual testing ground to affirm her lovability and desirability. The fascination with romance, then, becomes misused, misguided. Diana and others like her project themselves too energetically into the heroine's role, asking only to be transported to a state of happiness by being swept away. They want to escape the harsh realities of life through these romantic interludes, but this kind of romance does not last. Life has a way of taking over. The rent must be paid; problems must be solved.

When we try to live out romantic fantasies by

encouraging someone to "take care of us," when our pleasure stems from breathlessly surrendering our lives too easily to someone who fits the image of a hero, *beware*. Romance has a way of clouding perceptions. It becomes all too simple to favor powerlessness—giving oneself over to another—rather than self-control. Our belief in the value of romance, which is overstated and overblown, should never be the deciding factor in choosing a man.

## From "I" to "We"

Marriage is complicated. Two people join together with the good intention of creating continuity, a family, a balanced life. Within this framework, a woman's personality and focus can change. She gets an inkling of the change when she hears herself saying things (or discovers herself doing things) that would have been out of character years before. She can ignore the implications, but it usually means that she has begun to think in terms of "we" instead of "I" and "him." The "I" to "we" change is not based on altruism. Rather, it's a blurring of separateness between husband and wife. "I" gets lost, "we" takes over, and a woman becomes a wife in the most stereotypical way—because the "I" that gets lost most often is hers, not the man's. That's when many marriages go from "I do" to "I don't."

"Who am I?" these women ask me. "How did I lose myself along the way?" It might have been romance that got them into the marriage in the first place (as in Diana's case) or the assumption that they would be cared for, tended, protected (Martha's story). There's an expensive trade-off when a woman lives for a man and becomes a functionary in his life while being afraid to do anything that will risk his displeasure.

What are the qualities that tamper with individuality within marriage? Teri McCormick, the producer of my television show in Detroit, was once speculating about factors that turn a woman into a wife—the blending of "I" into "we" that eventually goes from "I do" to "I don't."

"I think it begins," Teri says, "when the woman will not be fair to herself and to her husband. She has unrealistic expectations about marriage and a belief in certain myths that trap her." These myths are worth looking at.

*He'll be different after marriage.* This is chancy thinking. Few men change within marriage, though they will relax personal habits. (He won't be as natty as he was when calling for you on a date, but instead will be happy in a creased T-shirt.) Nevertheless, he *told* you that he'd make changes. Before marriage, for example, he may have promised that things would be different after you took your vows. He may have assured you that his spending habits would be different. With the incentive of marriage, he wouldn't gamble, spend so freely, be such a good pal and lend cash so freely. Or, after marriage, he wouldn't be living alone any longer and won't need to drink as much—he'd soon have you by his side to calm him down.

When we go from "I" to "we" in this trap, we step beyond agreeing with his fantasies and enter into them with conviction. Whatever objectivity we may have had about his promises, whatever doubts we harbored that those promises were false, are lost to the dream of his changing—his changing for *us*. In truth, it may be the *woman* who's different.

Now that she's a wife, her patterns must conform to her image of wifeliness; in turn, she thinks her husband must be her ideal spouse, the man who will act on his word. She assigns him a role, or many roles—he's provider, lover, confidant, her everything. If he's always had it in him, he will fulfill her expectations. If not, he will always be the same man who placed the ring on her finger, and more so.

*It is most important to recognize about your chosen man that what you see is what you get.* Be aware of who he is and tune in to that, not a dream of him. Don't be tempted to fall in love with a man's *potential* rather than the *reality* of what he is. And leave the rehabilitation to the social workers.

*To be a good wife, she's got to say yes.* Another expectation tells us that it is our duty to go from "I" to "we." Deferential behavior is the rule. A wife's ideas are rarely subjects for discussion within her four walls. Instead, she asks permission: *"Can I . . . ?"* Her husband may agree or not, but she is subjected to psychological pressure as she worries over his answer. If a marriage has been set up so that the wife must ask permission, she should ask herself why she has pulled back and allowed someone else to make the decisions. Why is she so passively participating in her own life? Why is she inviting a hard case of resentment that may eventually lead her from "I do" to "I don't"?

It's easy for some women to immerse themselves in this myth and lose that sense of "I." They believe that the more they give a husband, the more they agree with him, the more he's pleased, the more they'll get in return—even if their wishes have yet to be granted.

There's the hope that if *they* keep saying yes, eventually *he'll* say yes. Unfortunately, this kind of husband is not usually interested in saying yes to his wife's needs. His interest lies in her acquiescence. He's perfectly comfortable with having his wife seek his approval.

This is a seriously imbalanced marriage, one with little spirit of true partnership. To make the marriage work, this wife must give 90 percent of herself over to her husband for 10 percent of his involvement. To her distress, this wife may find out too late that her husband will never fulfill her fantasy and accommodate himself to her needs or eagerly seek her opinions. What she'll have is a lifetime of yessing a man, living entirely for him.

*He'll want for us what we want for ourselves.* We may believe that a husband is anxious for our success, that he's a personal cheering squad who's as fascinated with our goals as we are. Many working women with ambitions soon discover that they are living with a man who once rooted for their success but now boos them down. He wanted her to succeed, all right, but only to the limit he had in mind. Not where she intended to go.

It's not uncommon for two-career couples to set up plans for the future. They may even draw up strategies for his advancement and ideas for hers. Sounds reasonable, but here's the snag: Career-oriented women often report they are working for "us," so "we" can have more money, a better life. They cannot reconcile their own pleasure in succeeding out there in the world, and swear their efforts are only for "us." The "I" may be doing her work, but "we" gets the credit.

Some husbands are unable to deal with wives who earn more or as much as they do or who hold an executive title they themselves covet. If she has too much money and too big a title, it may be unsettling for him. He didn't plan on having his wife skip ahead so briskly while he's still trudging uphill. But he remembers that she once worked for "us," losing just enough of herself in that original togetherness. Outdoing him—or equaling him—establishes her identity as an accomplished woman, and he may well be angry about it. He may turn on her, finding subtle or obvious ways to sabotage her success. He may be partially proud, but another part of him is outdone.

*He's a hero.* In his assigned role as master of your universe, he must know, intuit, judge, perform, command. He is the protector: He stands with his chest to the wind; we stand behind him, shielded and sheltered from the torrent. He is the lover: He must sense how to satisfy us sexually even if we don't give him a hint of what pleases us or what doesn't.

When we believe this myth, we give up "I" by placing a man in an exalted position. Since a hero doesn't make mistakes, he knows everything. Since a hero is invulnerable, he will protect us. A hero is also endowed with a complete understanding of human behavior, so his perceptions of others are always faultless. We defer to this demigod in a number of ways, and it comes out like this: "We," for example, have decided that he's to handle all the finances since he's so much more clever at juggling funds. (That is, you were perfectly capable of balancing a checkbook before you were married, but now he wants control of his money and yours.) "We" have decided to drop a friend who's a "bad influence" on you. (That is, you like her, but he's jealous of your attention to her, so she goes.)

What happens if the hero falls from grace? He not only fails himself, but us as well, and soon enough we start to see him as a failure. We gave ourselves over to a man we needed to be great, but he disappointed us. "We" didn't live up to expectations.

*Marriage is about happiness.* Only recently have expectations in marriage been attuned to personal fulfillment—to happiness as a goal. Marriages were once political and economic alliances that worked, when they worked, because it was a sacred agreement that also functioned in the spirit of partnership. Love was not mandatory before the ceremony, although out of those traditional marriages, it often did develop. I'm not suggesting a return to arranged marriages, rather that we can learn one thing from them—*make the marriage work.* And this success can produce real happiness—a mutual sharing and caring for each other.

Now, we may start out being in love, and because we do, we want to cling to that intensity. We know it does not last; love changes. So if happiness does not necessarily mean love in a marriage, what *does* it mean? *Marriage is a collaboration, a goal jointly sought.* Within this union happiness can be defined in many ways. A critical component of the definition should include that we are free to develop ourselves individually, and our partner is not an obstacle. When you cannot develop freely, or if a spouse is not giving you what you want, you are unhappy. You think marriage has failed you. Where did you go wrong?

Tracy Cabot wrote a book with an interesting theme; it's called *How to Make a Man Fall in Love With You.* In it she details strategies for arousing a man to love, the goal being his eventual proposal of marriage. "Tuning in" to him, she instructs, is crucial. ("Get him to talk about himself," our mothers coached us with similar advice when we began to date.) Mirror his gestures, Cabot further advises us—this comforts him

—and *breathe as he breathes*. She proceeds to let us in on how to acquire this secret. "You can tell how quickly a man is breathing by watching his shoulders. Mark them with a point on the wall behind him and watch them go up and down. Then simply start breathing yourself in the same rhythm."

If breathing when he breathes spurs him to love, what do we do when he moves away from the wall? What do we do years later when we are so resentful of him that we don't care if he's breathing at all? We may develop clever stratagems to win a man, but will he be the right man? It should not matter if we breathe in the same rhythm, although mastering the trick may amuse both of you for the moment. Give a man complete power (you *are* if you are coordinating your actions with his own) and he will not give up much of that power without a formidable battle. Breathe as he breathes and you may soon be gasping for breath. Breathe as he breathes and he will expect you to be a part of him. To him, your marriage made the two of you "we." That "we" is him.

If you set up too rosy a picture of how marriage will bring you happiness by first making him happy, you are creating the kind of situation that will take you from "I do" to "I don't." Why? Under these circumstances, your happiness can never count for as much as his does. This realization can be shattering. A marriage weighted in a man's favor cannot fulfill both partners. Breathe as *you* breathe . . .

These myths and expectations may be responsible for your disappointment in marriage, but all is not lost. You can still retrieve good feelings with a spouse and reconstruct a marriage. For many of us, going from "I do" to "I don't" and back to "I do" is a real possibility.

# Going Back to "I Do"

Going from "I do" to "I don't" and back to "I do" is all about learning to change fears into challenges—within and without marriage—and how to establish a balance where *you can be* and can *love and let be*.

Going from "I don't" back to "I do" implies that you are dissatisfied with a life in imbalance. If you are alone, it can mean opening up and taking another in. It's knowing that work enriches the soul, but that work can pulse with greater intensity when there is a personal life around it. In marriage, imbalance can be exhausting—you live for another's comfort, regulate time by another's needs. Instituting a balance means you must find a way to establish and express *your* needs, too, and have them respected.

Going from "I do" to "I don't" and back to "I do" implies that you have embraced one guiding philosophy—to love and let be. Disappointed expectations get in the way of harmony. One of these expectations is "having it all"—marriage, children, successful career, community prominence, a country home on some golden shore. Having it all sounds glamorous, perfect. It marks a woman as capable, exceptional, caring—a brilliant engineer of life. For the married careerist, failing to have it all can be as crushing as for the married woman who's afraid to take the first steps toward applying for a job, or the single woman who is unable to say yes to marriage. Is having it all worth the struggle?

Letty Cottin Pogrebin remarks in *Family Politics* that "having it all means *adding* roles, not altering those we already play with such difficulty. If having it all really was a new frontier of freedom (i.e., more is better), men would want *in* on nurturing, preparing food and staying home. But that's not what 'all' means. It doesn't mean men doing more, it means 'letting' women do what men do without changing what men do."

Having it all will take its toll on those who are not prepared to deal with the consequences. We *are* adding roles. We cannot all be Geraldine Ferraro, run for public office, and have our teenage daughter quote for the press, "My parents are so much in love, it's disgusting." To have it all, you must be able to divide your life into smaller segments and let everyone know that when you are with them, it must *count*. If you are lucky, you have a husband who will not punish you for having an absorbing career, and your children will already have learned from your example that hard work, caring behavior and independence aren't such a bad combination. Pogrebin is right—men don't want any part of loading the washer. But what we need to do within marriage is help a husband increase his satisfaction in the choices we've made by letting him know they can benefit *him* too. Many women, at various stages of their lives, confront this problem. You may recognize your situation from among these examples.

   • You are single, involved in a rewarding career and find a certain comfort in it. Now it's happened—an inner tug toward marriage. You are someone who nearly has it all, but without a man. You worry about what will happen if you marry. Understandably, many women fear that they will make a man the center and core of their lives, and thus be forced to sacrifice their careers.
   • You are a woman who wants children after many years of marriage, reversing a long-standing

decision not to have them. How will children fit into your life? Can you have children after all, since you're getting closer to forty or are over forty? How will a child affect the relationship with your husband, your career?

• You are a woman who's never worked, but your kids are all in school and you're bored. You want a career, or at least a job that occupies mind, heart and hands. Without productive work, life has come to feel empty. Where can you find a job? What can you do? How far can you go?

• You are a woman who's opted to leave home to find your identity. Yours has been a restrictive marriage. Married to a thumbs-down kind of man, you feel you must leave to "be," to free yourself. Your husband is excessively controlling, monitoring, and approving or disapproving of your every action.

• You are a woman who seriously wants or intends to leave her marriage because you are emotionally unfulfilled, abused; you have nothing in common with your husband. On the one hand, you have trouble leaving. If you can't end the marriage yet, it's because uprooting a life you've helped structure is difficult, painful. You give yourself reasons to stay—you need a family even if it's only a semblance of one. Conversely, you've decided to leave and discover that although fearful of the future, you feel relief about going. As a woman on the way out of her marriage, you don't tamper with certain incendiary topics. Your husband is drinking again, for example. At last you don't have to say, "Haven't you had enough?" Why fall into the same old trap? You don't need to. One day you know the marriage is over—not when he makes you furious, but when he doesn't.

All these reservations about changing the status of your marriage (or venturing into marriage) are valid— but they needn't be considered as cataclysmic events. When you think they are, the associated feelings of "I don't" take over. The first thought is that you've selected the wrong man, the very one who cannot "understand" you.

I wish I could pluck the right man for the right woman out of the crowd. Since I can't, I'd like to give you this instead: If you are ready for the perfect man, the union will be joyous, miraculous—but not without conflict. Conflict is built into marriage the way a pit is built into a cherry. We must learn to be smart cookies and keep what we have of value. We must learn that marriage is a business arrangement with deeper feeling —but a business relationship nevertheless. We must learn not to let a marriage slip through our fingers and then ask innocently, "How come other people have happy marriages and I don't?" Smart cookies will take responsibility for their share of the marriage.

There are a number of ideals connected with taking a marriage back to "I do." Ideally, marriage is where you find peace—a comment that Jane Fonda made about her relationship with her husband, Tom Hayden: "Marriage is where you're free to say, I really don't feel like talking right now, without worrying if the other person will accuse you of selfishness." When you can communicate ideally, you have the ability to say, "I want to be held, I don't want sex." Ideally, marriage is where you can speak openly to your husband. Ideally, it's a place where you can face, hard as it may be, what *you* are doing to contribute to whatever conflicts exist. Can you see how you set up situations to bait him, get a rise out of him, express jealousy—just to affirm your power? Ideally, within marriage, you are still attracted to each other physically. Ideally, you can talk openly about what bothers you and not let things slip fifteen years down the line. Holding grudges serves only to keep an emotional and divisive distance.

Ideally, we can love and let be.

—But we can also *love and let go* if it's necessary.

"We would have broken up except for the children," said comedian Mort Sahl of his marriage. "Who were the children? Well, she and I were." Profoundly said with a hilarious edge—and so true. Why do we leave? Why do we stay? What reasons do women reach for?

For some, it's because their husbands are passive and don't make decisions. But if you make the choices and he goes along with them, you get to live life your way with an amiable companion. If he's generous enough to go along with it, accept this bounty! Love and let be: this man will be forever passive about decision making until he is ready to be decisive, not before. You're then on your way back to "I do."

A woman tells me that her husband has serial affairs and she wants out of the marriage. I'd say: Look to see if it's solely his problem or a problem between the two of you. What do the affairs offer him that your relationship doesn't? You needn't pry out details about the other woman (blond? thin? smart? dumb? gushily approving of him?)—this will cause you pain. Just ask: What does she have for him? Do you lack this quality? Can you retrieve it if you once had it? Is your husband happy to come home and get back into his marriage—never mind the affairs? If he is, your marriage may still be worth saving and you can get back on the road to "I do."

A wife tells me her husband demonstrates no interest in the children. He will not play with them, care for them even for short periods or spend time getting to know them. Looking deeper into the situation, I found that she holds the children too close to her, making her husband feel excluded, estranged. The children are not only *hers*, occupying her world, but they are also her allies against him. She spends so much of her energy winning the children's affection, often resorting to talking against her husband, that they feel uncomfortable with him. She simply needs to include him in his own family. Then "I do" can follow naturally.

These examples offer a few ideas for turning a marriage around. It isn't easy to do—I know that. But the first step is telling the truth about the relationship. It's not only a matter of pointing out his problems, but also of accepting your own and understanding what the marriage means.

To reach a satisfactory state of "I do," you'll need to scrutinize your marriage by honestly answering the questions posed in the next section.

# Where Is Your Marriage Now?

What is your marriage all about right now?

Could you go back and look at what attracted you to the man you chose? What were his good qualities? Did you choose him to complete yourself? Did he fail to complete yourself? Did he fail to complete you and himself over the years? Do you feel you've grown more than he has?

What follows is a series of questions to help you figure out where you are in your marriage. Articulate as best you can what you expect from yourself and your husband. Do your answers reflect dreams that you should have outgrown years ago? In 1983, *Ladies' Home Journal* conducted an interesting survey called

"The Portrait of the American Woman Today." Nearly 90,000 readers responded. The survey asked women about their feelings as wives, workers, mothers. The section on marriage noted this: After citing financial problems as being the first to create discord in marriages ("love won't pay the rent"), respondents said they yearned for more communication, both verbal and physical. A good percentage said that while they respect old values, they've come to embrace some of the *new* values in terms of, for example, a husband's greater participation in child care.

The survey concluded: "The modern woman's marriage is one in which she and her husband seem to be making up rules as they go along, without any proven models to guide them in their choices." Women are in transition, therefore marriage is in transition. We need to clarify what works for us and build, if not a proven model for others, *proof* that marriage can work by putting in some effort. Yours and his. Answering these questions will help you in that effort.

- Why did you marry?
- How did you expect things would change between you and your husband?
- What did you think would be different about your life?
- What did you want him to do for you beyond what you'd already done for yourself?
- What were you interested in doing for him?
- What obligations did you expect him to undertake? Has he?
- What obligations did he expect from you?
- Did you want to pool your money or keep separate accounts?
- Did you discuss careers? What if you get a

promotion and he doesn't so you wind up earning more than he does?

• Did you discuss having children?

• If he was previously married, did you openly discuss his obligations to his first wife and children?

• If you were previously married and have children, did you discuss his role with your children?

• Did you discuss who would be the disciplinarian with your children?

• Did you want to have a family with him and why—though both of you already have children from previous marriages?

• Did you talk about what will happen if the feelings you have for each other change?

• Have you talked about having or not having outside relationships? Does it come as a surprise when your spouse is unfaithful?

• Are you willing to make certain compromises and sacrifices, such as not being able to just take off and go somewhere without calling home first? Do you resent checking in?

• Has he made a declaration that his relationship with you comes before all others, including his mother, father, and siblings?

• Did he expect you to take up where he left off caring for his parents, so you must do it?

• Did you have to follow his parents' rules and let them make decisions about your life?

• Have you talked about dealing with sexual refusals so neither of you feels rejected, hurt or angry?

• How do you decide where to take vacations?

• What are the things that being married to him will enhance in your life?

• Do you feel a genuine sense of friendship, is he

willing to accept changes as you grow? Are you changing just to please him?

• Does your husband feel proud of you—that he's gotten a prize?

• Is he interested in sharing all the important parts of his life with you—how much he makes, what he feels?

• Are you each other's confidant?

• Can you stand toe to toe with him and offer an honest opinion when he asks for it?

• Do you feel that he is so superior to you in a number of ways that you are in awe of him?

• Are you afraid to hear his criticism of you?

• Can he tease you without being destructive?

• Is he a soulmate to share the adventure of life?

Reflect carefully on these questions. It might strike you that the answers you give now are ones you might not have given years before—especially during the first two years of marriage. That's okay. Your perceptions may have changed as your goals changed. Your marriage has evolved, and, interestingly, you've evolved. "How did I get here?" you ask. "Who would have guessed that . . . ?" "If I had only known that. . . ."

Few of us "know." Life just isn't that predictable. Every woman faces the possibility of death, divorce or desertion of a spouse. That is why I urge women not to leave marriages that still hold a chance for growth *toward* each other, not *from* each other. But if marriage becomes more a matter of pain than pleasure, leaving may be the only answer. If it happens, it's not the end at all, but a new challenge to face. And the challenge will be to get *better,* not *bitter.*

# 6

## Don't Get Bitter, Get Better

At fifty years old, Lily Ann Grossman Ravitch is enjoying her life. She divorced at forty-eight after twenty-eight years of marriage. "I could honestly say we were best friends for most of our marriage," she said. "My husband and I just outgrew each other. I was the one who asked for the divorce, and it took him by surprise."

Lily Ann, president of InDepth Diet Counseling and International Diet Centers and manufacturer's representative for a building materials company, is a dynamic, enthusiastic woman who would not allow bitterness to enter into any aspect of that growing apart within marriage. "Until the end, we showed respect and love for each other. Our marriage had pretty much been one of mutual kindness. Divorcing, miraculously, didn't change things."

Her ex-husband married very soon after the divorce. "It was a compliment," Lily Ann said cheerfully. "He'd come from a good marriage. Why wouldn't he want another one?"

Fifteen years ago, Lily Ann began to stretch beyond

her role of wife and mother. She went into business and began to succeed. "My ex-husband is a traditional man—he prefers his wife at home. I knew it bothered him, even threatened him, but I had to make that job work for me. He told me plaintively a number of times, 'I want my little wife back.' That was no longer me," she said.

Work filled her life after the divorce. She dated, but "I didn't think I needed a husband. I was almost fifty—and the strength I felt being alone was a revelation. I was okay on my own. Then I met a man quite casually through friends. What happened, exactly, I don't know, but we fell in love within days! I never expected it, but three months later, we married."

This marriage is different for her. "We're both at a point in life where we can be independent and want to be together. I'm my own person, working, loving it. My husband has his life, his business. It's a matter of maturity, I think. Reaching out when you need help, reaching out to find what's best for you, and reaching out to others. When you do, you discover you're more accomplished than you think you are."

Lily Ann's story inspires me, and I tell it to you for this reason: Over the last ten years or so, I've encountered very few married women who have not been bitter about what marriage has wrought. But Lily Ann is someone who is not bitter. Why is she different? She started out as we all did—with dreams of marital glory. Dreams fade hard. What happened? Our expectations going into marriage were not just vividly optimistic, they were dazzlingly idealistic. In each other's arms we were a team, miraculously in love, seeking happiness, sure that we could endure mountains of travail. But the business of life is harsh, and romance has never been much of a survival technique. Sorrowfully, 50 percent of those kindred souls will leave us or be left by us—we, the women who once believed this man would complete our lives. We damn ourselves as unlucky.

Divorce is rupturing. Painful. Lawyers fight lawyers on behalf of the two former soulmates, sometimes over the possession of something as unimportant as a set of paring knives. Children are torn between loyalties to the warring parents. One spouse sends the other a bill for taking the children to dinner and demands reimbursement. Divorce is not a pretty sight. It can mark us, make us bitter, disoriented, caught in an emotional and financial limbo.

Failed marriages share a number of characteristics, and having unrealistic expectations is certainly among the most common in claiming the disillusioned. And the most unrealistic expectation of all is that a man will bring to a woman all that is good in life. Clinging to that expectation during the early years of marriage, a woman casts a blind eye toward the problems and flaws in a relationship. Insecurities are closer to the surface during those first two years of learning about each other. The young bride hesitates to bring up an issue, positive that by doing so she will irrevocably disturb whatever harmony there is, as well as extinguish passion. Communication problems during those exploratory years are often solved not by discussion and action, but by having sex. The pleasure covers up issues and, incidentally, feeds them—the issues grow plumper by the year until even lovemaking, no matter how spectacular, suffers along with everything else.

Any woman reading this should shudder if there's an issue she can't discuss with her husband to make life better for both of them.

Just as we have been taught to have unrealistic

expectations about marriage—"From I Do to I Don't" introduced you to some of them—so have we been taught to cling to the nest rather than risk the voyage out. Solo flights are not for everyone. Often, though, the nest is cluttered with grudges, hurts, replays of the same arguments, pat summaries of life. Over the years, bitterness mounts, especially for the homemaker who doesn't have the resources to confront the issues that matter to her. Along the way, there may be a blurring of identity and she may lose herself in her husband's image. After a while, it's hard for her to identify herself as a separate individual. When the marriage ends, she's nothing, she thinks, without him.

Here we are concerned about what remains in your cycle of life after the disruption of divorce, and how to combat bitterness in spite of your history. If you are suddenly thrust into the world, you need time to get your bearings, keep your life in some sort of gratifying shape. No one recovers from divorce overnight. What you want to do is wake up with some enthusiasm as you enter a new phase of life. You can build a new world without the man who was once your entire world, and I ask that you do it without bitterness. I ask you to get better for your own sake. If you are contemplating divorce, what you are reading may help you decide to stay in your marriage and renew yourself within its boundaries.

Of all the qualities most evident in women when they describe their unhappy marriages, it is bitterness that most affects them. It shapes the form of marriage after a while, and lingers on after the divorce. Hundreds of women have spoken to me about such bitterness, and I want to tell you some of their stories and how they coped by way of example. Perhaps you will see a piece of your own life within these tales and learn how to change your marriage around just enough to remake it into a union of mutual trust and friendship.

Lily Ann's secret, if there is one, is *faith in herself* coupled with a basically optimistic disposition. Unfortunately, her opposites abound—women without a thread of hope or self-confidence. Vivian is one, a strikingly pretty woman I know who, after eight years of being tortured by divorce is exhausted from the energy she puts into perpetuating inertia.

As she will quickly admit, Vivian married her Prince Charming "for all the wrong reasons"—he was a smooth-talking, handsome, prosperous young man, but a womanizer, a high roller. Vivian was in love.

After a twenty-year tempestuous marriage, Greg left her. He'd always been unfaithful, uncommunicative, and finally saw no point in staying with her any longer. His parting tirade revealed his twenty years' worth of bitterness—before that she was unable to coax much out of him. They'd communicated by arguments, insults and eventual apologies for unresolved problems. He delivered his parting dig coldly: he told her that his father had picked her out for him and that he'd never loved her. A shattering revelation to accept, and Vivian was even more appalled to discover that her husband had told their daughter that he wanted a divorce before even telling her.

Greg's lawyers were smarter than hers; she was not given much in the way of alimony and had to get a job. The catch-22 was that she was working when Greg left, but was told by her lawyer to quit so she could get more alimony, but it didn't work that way at all. Alone, in her mid-forties, she felt she couldn't compete with younger women for the available men—"I was too old, didn't have money and couldn't play tennis, in that order," she says. Vivian stayed at home, under her blankets. After some prodding, she took a few courses, but stopped, convinced a certificate wouldn't lead to a gratifying job. She wallows in her despair as completely as her husband did in his selfishness, bitterly blaming him and blocking the changes that might make her better.

It is sad for me to see the Vivians of this world who resist getting better. Bitterness is nonproductive, wasteful, all too easy to slip into. Misery doesn't require plans or goals, and it leads nowhere. It's here to be conquered, though. Let's take a closer look.

# Bitterness: Where Does It All Start?

A patient describes a moment to me that changed her life. She was paring apples late at night to make a pie for a dinner party the following day. Her husband was watching TV in the next room, or, rather, Josh was restlessly hitting the buttons every few seconds. It was an ordinary scene from their married life together, no different from other days spent not quite in each other's company, but much more significant. It was at that moment that Susan knew she wanted out of her marriage but did not know how she could survive the breakup. The revelation chilled her to the quick.

Marriages dissolve at the astonishing rate of one every twenty-seven seconds. Right then, Susan could understand why. The marriage never seemed to be working out, but she'd always had hopes. Everyone has hopes. What went wrong? When she met Josh, she'd been mesmerized by passion, the "chemistry" between them, the need to stop time so the bliss wouldn't end with the start of a new day. He was more than Susan ever expected to have, even temporarily, in her life.

Eight years before, Susan was Josh's secretary; his wife at the time was a petite blonde who loved staying home to care for their children—all four of them.

Then there was Susan—sultry, available and tantalizing to Josh. To Susan, Josh represented the height of gratifying love packaged in a person who was also financially successful—her image of the perfect man. A torrid affair decided Josh on his next move: he'd leave his wife and family and marry Susan.

Josh could not handle the crisis of divorce and remarriage, as Susan learned within six months. He continues to deny Susan children while he overindulges his own. During the last six of their eight years of marriage, Josh has become less and less interested in sex—though it was that immeasurable craving for each other that led to their union. Susan's presence reminds Josh that he broke up his first family and that he cannot reconcile himself to creating a second one with the woman he deems "responsible" for his torment. Instead of leaving Susan, he verbally abuses her. "He calls me a whore on every possible occasion," she told me. "It destroys me because what have I ever done but want him?" I asked her to explain further.

"He *married* me," she continued, "and I thought that would be the answer to everything. I didn't want to hurt his ex-wife, but I felt she'd be okay. They didn't have a marriage anyway, just the pretext of one. Josh is simultaneously suffering feelings of guilt toward her, and obligation toward me, like a contract he can't break. I feel locked into this relationship, too, tortured by some similar sense of obligation. Both of us would be happier elsewhere—Josh back with his first wife and kids, me alone, far away from civilization with nothing but peace, quiet, no Josh, no men, no marriage, no terror."

One evening when Susan least expected it—eight years down the line—the symptoms hit, and hit with a stunning clarity. It was the moment of saturation— she'd had enough. It was a moment of anger for having taken abuse for so long. It was a moment of knowing she could save her life by leaving, but she believed she'd die if she took the first step toward the door. It was a moment followed by bitterness.

Sometimes you will, as Susan did, experience the symptoms of bitterness all at once and know what it will mean to you a bit further down the line: there may be a divorce because you see no resolution other than dissolving the marriage. Or you hang in there with the unresolved issues while hoping for relief and change, but feeling sure things will remain the same. As time passes, you are coolly clear about these points: You are happier alone than when a glance at the clock tells you that your husband is on his way home. When he *is* home, *you* yearn not to be. Each day you may feel that your life isn't enhanced by him; that he detracts from it or makes no difference one way or the other. You find reasons to avoid coming home, delaying simple confrontations. Or, when you hear his key in the door and your body quickens, every muscle clenches—you know an argument will follow very shortly. You look for reasons not to have sex with him, or overdress for bed. You don't fill him in on family gossip or casual anecdotes. Why bother?

You want him to change, you wish there were a way to re-win the marriage to the way it was when it was at its peak. You repeat to youself over and over, *How did this marriage happen to me?* Being at odds with the man whom you expected to fulfill you suddenly appears

190

incomprehensible. This was not what you expected of marriage, of yourself, of the man who fathered your children, who once knew how to have a good time in your company, who once respected you.

For most women, bitterness grows from a profoundly similar source—shattering disappointment in the course of their lives, along with an accompanying feeling of powerlessness to alter what pains them. Susan overvalued the torrid love between her and Josh and what it could accomplish. She discovered that for her, the hottest love was outside marriage; inside marriage she was punished for the same ardor. Vivian, wretchedly unhappy as she huddles under her blankets, prefers a daily dose of bitter brews of her own making. Bitterness controls her and has controlled her for eight years. She loathes her life, but she desperately wants a man to share in the life she hates. She can't stand to be alone on Saturday night, yet she wants someone to be with her for a lifetime.

Both these women were disappointed in the men they chose and how they were treated by them. Other women suffer from bitterness in other ways; let's take a look at the lessons that can be learned from their stories.

# The Bitterness of Dwelling on the Past

Bitterness grows when we can't make peace with what we've lost and enjoy what has taken its place. In Sarah's story, you can see how she impulsively disconnected from what could have been a better life. Married young to a charming young doctor, Sarah discovered that her looks were enough to interest her husband before marriage, but later he demanded a more sparkling intellectual companionship. Sarah was intimidated by Dan and couldn't keep pace with him. Miserably unhappy after four years of marriage and one child, she wanted out. Her parents pretty much planned her getaway while Dan was at the hospital one day—she took everything with her. Back in her parents' home, she knew she'd made a dreadful mistake by leaving in a panic. At twenty-five, she thought her life was over. Resigned, Sarah got a job as a bookkeeper and raised her child.

Nine years later, she was introduced to a handsome widower with a teenage daughter. Mack ran a gas station, spoke street English and had barely gotten out of the eighth grade, but he was kind, loved Sarah and wanted to marry her. At thirty-seven she had his daughter.

Sarah is now sixty and she asks herself, is it too late to change? From the age of twenty-five, she remained bitter over the dissolution of her first marriage—the one that could have been ideal. In her memory, she was beautiful and a man of worth valued her; Dan was brilliant and ambitious. They were the perfect couple. She could have been a revered doctor's wife. But Dan encouraged her feelings of intellectual inadequacy, and she took it to mean she wasn't good enough for him, for his position, in any way. She panicked and fled. She regrets that divorce now when she looks across the table at unshaven Mack, resenting him for not being a polished gentleman, for not conferring glory on her. Insecure in who she was, Sarah longed to be raised to a higher level of public esteem through someone else—a doctor. Perhaps she didn't love Dan for himself in the first place, but for what he might do for her. When there was no payoff, she packed up and left too quickly. She spent the years of her second marriage wrathful toward Mack, unappreciative of him and any caring gesture he made; nothing was enough.

But something clicked with Sarah at sixty and she began observing herself within her relationships. She wanted something better for the remainder of her life. Possibly she realized that her children didn't like being with her, that her husband tried to avoid her company, that her sisters rattled off litanies of excuses for not visiting her. She'd locked herself into a "tragedy"—the loss of her young doctor—and let it create her life. Past middle age, how many more years did she have? she asked herself. She did not want to live them this way. Not anymore. But could she change?

There comes a point in the maturation of a person's character when, like Sarah, you travel down a road and reach a fork. If you continue down the same old road, there will be more misery—no positive payoffs, no pleasure, no growth. "I admit it," she tells me. "I made a terrible mistake. I picked one wrong husband and made myself and others suffer. Can I start over?"

# The Bitterness of Unrealistic Hope

Too many women cannot accept it when their husband leaves, secretly waiting for his return because they're sure he will, bitter when he doesn't. I heard about Rhonda through a friend. Rhonda is thirty-eight, was married for six years, separated for four, and has been divorced for three years. When Tom first filed for divorce, Rhonda was a veteran of four years of separate living, but it did not prepare her for what she knew was coming. Instead, she denied it. Tom could not really mean to divorce her, she wanted to believe. When he left years before, she told all who would listen that it was merely a trial separation. Tom moved in immediately with another woman. This didn't disturb Rhonda —another woman wasn't evidence enough that Tom wanted out of their marriage. For four years she called Tom two or three times a week, sure she could win him back. Tom was a traditional man who required an enormous amount of attention. Rhonda played on this, checking in with him, offering her services, even listening to a few of Tom's complaints about the woman he was living with. Rhonda held on to her belief that he would return.

Tom intended to marry his girlfriend, but first he had to divorce Rhonda. The news of the divorce devastated her. She'd waited four years for Tom to return, but he had other plans. She'd been his pal, made few demands, and for her trouble was served with divorce papers. Rhonda feels bitter, betrayed, undone, outdone. "I thought I knew him," she wails. On the one hand, though Rhonda knew she had been rejected by Tom, she persisted in being available, forgiving, waiting out what was perhaps a fling. She insinuated herself into his life without disrupting Tom's new relationship —she assumed the pose of a very modern woman. The initial rejection was intolerable, but she didn't want to hate him and she was so sure they'd be reconciled. "I wanted him in my life in some way," she explains. "I didn't want to share him, but I couldn't lose him. I was willing to wait till he tired of her, for the phase to pass."

And on the other hand? Rhonda couldn't face the truth—that Tom was gone. In her fantasy, Tom would reject the other woman when he realized whom he'd

left behind—the devoted woman who'd wait for years
—and forgive him. She knew her man, she thought.
Hadn't she always taken care of him? Why stop?

What Rhonda tallies up now is four lost years waiting
for Tom and three more of mourning her ineptitude
because her mission failed. And she's bitter. Wasn't she
the understanding, sacrificing wife? How many women
can listen to a husband talk about problems with his
mistress—and be sympathetic?

Orthodox marriage vows remind us that "till death us
do part," but we must recognize, painful though it may
be, that each of us has *the right* to leave, and that we
have the obligation to ourselves to rebuild a life without
the other. This is not to say that Rhonda should not
have waited, given him some time, but her investment
was far too costly. There is waiting with a purpose and
waiting to *give* your life purpose. Consumed with Tom,
Rhonda's life was constructed around their phone calls,
her driving by his apartment late at night, the persistent
fantasy that he was, and always would be, her husband.
All her energy and concentration went into winning
Tom back, and she has nothing to show for it but
bitterness.

# The Bitterness of Fearing Others' Opinions

Women who stay in an unhappy marriage because
they are overly concerned with what others will think if
they divorce are doomed to bitterness. Here's Joanna,
in her early thirties, with one child and a career in
advertising that's begun to take off. Joanna's marriage
is similar to many unions during these last fifteen years

or so—the formerly dependent wife goes out to work to supplement the family income and discovers herself to be the more resourceful moneymaker, the more ambitious partner of the two. Result: a husband who held the dominant position when his wife was a young, insecure working mother, is now threatened. He wants her as she was, not as she is becoming.

"No matter that today many men know differently," Lillian B. Rubin wrote wisely in *Intimate Strangers,* "that in their heads they understand that a woman's independence is at least as likely to enhance a marriage as to threaten it. The heart has other concerns." And so it does for Mark, Joanna's husband.

He's putting pressure on Joanna to "give the family more time," his way of discouraging her from immersing herself more energetically in corporate life. Joanna feels confident she could make it without Mark, but panics when she thinks of divorce. She's outgrown Mark, plainly and simply. She's still fond of him, but she feels their marriage can go nowhere, while Mark holds on to values contrary to her own. She's angry that she can't leave, and worried that when she's fifty she'll regret not having left.

What holds Joanna in this marriage where her bitterness multiplies daily? It's fear of the opinion of others that possesses her. *What will people think?* She frets that Mark, free of her, will be fair game for her single friends. She does not want him, but neither does she want him to be wanted by other women. She worries that married friends will feel superior to her. She accuses herself of being unable to hold a husband, of not being "feminine" enough, clever enough, lovable enough.

Living by and for what others think is a dangerous business. Whom do you please first? Yourself? Others?

*The greatest problem for women like Joanna is resistance to working to make her life better.* Joanna and Mark should either see a counselor and try to reconcile their values and needs so that she can live within the marriage, or Joanna must search her heart to see if this marriage really is doomed. Or she can accept the fact that it is already doomed. Excuses about "others" merely delay action: there's no way to change what they think. They already have opinions about her marriage. Those who care will stick by you; you are well rid of those who are indifferent.

# The Bitterness of Blaming

Bitterness is often the result when you blame your husband for everything that's gone sour in the marriage and won't look at what you may have contributed to the discord. How difficult it is for women to face this fact. I know how painful it can be when you feel abused and wronged and are then asked to acknowledge that you may have been a participant in maintaining the status quo or provoking the difficulties.

Remember, the blamer cannot believe she has any power. Everything that happens to her must be the result of outside forces exerted upon her. You walk into a room and ask her a question while she is pouring milk into a glass; the glass tips over and it's "your fault." The cure is often just a simple matter of seeing life beyond her own fingertips and allowing others *their* weaknesses, needs, desire for self-expression. But the silent blamers become pacifiers—they will do anything, arrange their lives in any suitable fashion, to make their man stay.

Unlike the blamer, who openly voices her views ("If

it wasn't for you, I'd be happy"; "Of course I got lost again—you can never give me the right directions"), the silent blamer keeps such accusations to herself. She may be thinking that another is to blame for her unhappiness or confusion, but she's too afraid to come right out and say so. She fears the consequences—at worst, her husband will leave her if she tells him what's bothering her; at the very least, he won't like her or will humiliate her in some way.

While all that resentment seethes within her, she presents to her husband the picture of a perfect, accommodating wife. She's submissive, pacifying his doubts, irritations, and fears in any way she can to keep him with her. Although she may blame him for what's gone wrong in the marriage and in her life, she works to maintain the status quo—even if it's merely the illusion of a good marriage. Her husband may never get more than a hint that she's dissatisfied. How could he when she sugar-coats the problems and eases *his* mind?

A patient, Dee, told me that her husband said he wanted out of their marriage after twenty-four years. This hurt her deeply, but she approached the breakup with dignity and presence of mind. "I didn't want him to stay if he found life so unbearable. Our marriage had been on the edge of collapse for about a year, and I did everything I could think of to sugar-coat it, make it a version of marriage I thought would tantalize him. I didn't want to hear that he didn't love me, so I did anything to get approval. We tried not to be alone together too often. I asked for his advice in my little-girl tone of voice—advice he knew I didn't need and that he begrudged giving me anyway. Name it, I did it—everything but accept that the marriage really had little going for it but my desperation and his obligations. He said he wanted to go, and though it hurt, I could only say, 'Richard, I'll miss you.' More than anything I would not beg him to stay. If he didn't want me in his life, I didn't want me in his life either."

Few of us are like Dee, able to level with a man in quite this manner. Go, she was telling him. I may not be able to give you my blessings, but I will not keep you against your will. A pacifier by conditioning, Dee discovered another resource within her when faced with a crisis—she was strong. To her surprise, it was less painful to finally hear from Richard that he wanted out than to go through more years of bitterness over his cruel indifference and icy politeness toward her excessive ministrations.

As women, we torture ourselves with fantasies about how much we give and how little the other does. It is often far worse to conjure up images of what you think will happen than to face the actual event. Only by facing the truth, facing your part in the scheme of things, can you go forward and cast off old habits—even blaming—and clear your mind and life for new opportunities.

Bitterness is elevated to such a significant position for some women because it becomes their power, focus, goal and career. Holding fast to bitterness, it is difficult to express much else. It shades all relationships—with a spouse, with children, friends, relatives, co-workers, the corner news dealer. Bitterness drenches us and we become soaked in self-pity. Bitterness will not bring a man back once he's decided to leave. Bitterness does not spite a husband. It only shows him that you cannot care about yourself and for yourself without him. You need not be bitter. Resist the temptation. In fact, a ceremony to close the relationship might be helpful. In a church or temple with close family and friends, you might allow yourselves a closing statement, one in which you both acknowledge that although you will no longer love each other and live together, you will work together to raise healthy children and to maintain a good memory of what you once had.

Divorce is a terrible sadness in our lives. All we can ask of ourselves after a decent period of mourning the death of the marriage is to keep an eye on the road ahead. It's false to believe that husbands all go merrily on to more while you are stuck with less. When he left or when you left him, he didn't take your life along with him. Your life is separate and distinct. You will need time to recover and turn your life around into startlingly new dimensions. Without bitterness.

# Some Truths about Marriage

There are a few truths I'd like to share with you that may help you be a smart cookie in your marriage. Keep them in mind.

## LUST VERSUS LOVE

There are people who are good lovers but not good people to love. The confusion between lust and love is most likely to occur in the romance of a first marriage. Desire is not the basis for a good marriage unless you anticipate that the romance will expire after about two years—which is when most statistics show that it just about fizzes out and the vicissitudes of life take over.

If you're romantically inclined, you tend to favor the

man who will complement you, complete you. You're gregarious; he's a hermit. You're thrifty; he's a gambler. You feel insecure in this world; he's all convincing bravado, spouting promises to care for you. The attraction of opposites may stir the fires of passion for a while, but the struggle for compatibility will result in a conflagration. Compatibility means facing the realities of the entire human condition, and romance is not primary. If you've matured, if that first romantic marriage has ended, you can go on to select a man more like yourself, but only if *you* like yourself. And he will be a man who enhances your life, who is attuned to your rhythms as you are to his. When you know the man is a good lover but not good to love, you can face the fact that the relationship may be over because you cannot live with him. Don't marry for sex and wonder why later on.

## SOMETIMES "REASONABLE" IS BETTER THAN "PERFECT"

Instead of searching for a *better* partner, or a *more perfect* partner, look for a *reasonable* partner. You are assured of greater success and satisfaction when you do. In some cases, applying this criterion may well save a marriage. Princes are superb—they smile a lot, but they expect to be served. If it's a prince, a superman or presidential material that you seek, you will have to work hard to keep him. The more reasonable partner may not be flashy, have clout or an international reputation, but he will be there for you at three in the morning. There may never be an individual who can share *every* part of your life or give you glamor, and that's okay. As a creative, thinking person, understand how you punish yourself by rejecting the man who might provide warmth, stability and continuity. As a converted romantic told me, "the greatest turn-on is compassion."

## IT'S NEVER TOO LATE

There's an ongoing myth that married folk have an intense sexual life, deep emotional commitment and a degree of measurable happiness as they nestle with their partners in bed at night. This is, to be blunt, nonsense. Many marriages consist of two strangers in a rowboat, gazing over each other's shoulders. Some exist with minimal sexual expression or satisfaction. Other couples are locked into perpetual misery or brutality and can't escape each other. The truth is that in 50 percent of marriages in America, people cohabit, pool money, share meals, and have minimal sexual and emotional attachments or enthusiastic caring. They glance at the other and think: "This is not what I expected. I want someone better, different, exciting, to make me feel alive again." So why do we look back on life with regret and bitterness and bemoan fate? Why the feeling of despair, as if marriage were a terminal disease?

Women often feel they've lost the best years of their lives in marriage, that it's too late to have a meaningful life or fulfill a fantasy. Take a moment and consider this: *Perhaps you didn't have any choice other than the one you made at the time.* Don't be bitter about it. A basic human error is to not take advantage of today but to live for "tomorrow." Time is irretrievable. Those years are gone, but you can start again as long as you have drive, a sense of adventure, a need for self-fulfillment, and one person willing to offer a hand and believe in you. That's all anyone needs—one loyal friend who may or may not be a spouse.

Women often ask me how I've gotten where I am. They want to achieve a measure of success, or their version of it, but believe they can't. I sympathize, but suggest a reappraisal of how we got to where we are, and what the possibilities may be. I was married young, had two small children; my husband was in medical school and I was obliged to work. It was soon clear to me that my ardor for work went beyond economics. I realized I needed more than the roles of wife and mother. Had I stayed home and duplicated my own mother's lifestyle as full-time homemaker, which was expected of me at the time, I'd have grown into a bitter woman because of the limitations set on me. Instead, I decided on specific goals and worked for them, sweated for them. It was hard work and tough on my family. So, for the woman who is my age—even younger or older—and is just starting out, I reply: We came from similar backgrounds, but I struck out on a different path at a time when that path wasn't for you. If this path is right for you now, seize the moment and start walking down it.

If hindsight is always accurate, and we're really smart cookies, we'll use what we've learned from our mistakes. Regrets and bitterness flourish when we do nothing about them. The French writer Colette said that it was one of the greater moments in life when you realize that you are not something, "but someone." To be someone, release yourself from bitterness, then plan and organize—even if it's a matter of mapping out a few days at a time. Doing nothing earns you nothing.

## LOVE AND LET GO

Bitterness is a maze of gloomy corridors; we can get lost within it, refusing to see the way out whether or not the door is flung open. The door *is* open. Step through it and you can begin to surrender bitterness and accept reality. This may be difficult to take in, but give it a try.

First, to love and let go, know that the pain you feel will linger for a while, turn into a mild ache, then become a memory. When you accept the divorce, you can start to set up a life free from emotional bitterness and stop resisting change and joy. When you are divorced *from* someone, not divorced *to* someone, you'll be able to love and let go.

It takes a special strength to love and let go. It comes from your needing to have the marriage end, finally end. It means that you're willing to risk saying to your husband, "I love you, but it's not enough," or, "I love you and I have to accept that you may leave," or, "I love you, but it's not good enough for either of us," or, "I feel you don't love me and I can't put any more energy into a relationship that goes nowhere and never will go anywhere."

## BUT LEAVE THE CHILDREN OUT OF IT!

When you love and let go, there is no paralysis from bitterness, from regrets, from building your own gloomy corridors in which to wander. But meet Judy, a woman still caught in a labyrinth of her own making—a woman who wants to take her children along with her on her voyage.

I was sitting in a restaurant with my husband and friends one evening when I spotted Judy across the room. She was with her ex-husband and three children, and everyone seemed to be enjoying one another's company. In fact, Judy was incandescent that night and seemed attentive toward her children and ex-husband. She spotted me, said something to her family and walked across the room to my table. Within seconds, Judy launched into a harangue about the activities at her table. She proceeded to denigrate her children for having a good time with that "blasted so-and-so," the bane of her existence, her accursed ex-husband, Todd.

When Judy was married to Todd, he was everything; she was nothing but his reflection. He left her, not for another woman, but for peace. Judy cannot forgive Todd for leaving her. She wants revenge, or at least the satisfaction of rejecting *him,* and she thinks her children should cooperate and cut him out of their lives. But why should they deny their father? At one point in her life, Judy thought enough of Todd to marry him, to have children with him. Now she wants them to hurt him. Meanwhile, she puts on a falsely cheerful front for him while speaking ill of him behind his back.

Bitterness affects your children, too. Nearly one third of American children do not live with both biological parents, and about half of all children of divorce can tell you that they haven't seen their fathers in a year. These are sad statistics. Fathers *do* disappear, desert families, create new ones and shun the first one they were responsible for. Todd is not one of these fathers, but Judy, in her bitterness, would prefer that he were.

If you hold a child too closely and demand collusion against the man who left you, you may not get the response you expected. Bitterness and damaging remarks have a way of boomeranging. A child can reason and defend her or his feelings for the parent who's left.

"He couldn't be that bad," one child told her mother. "He was smart enough to get away from you." When a mother speaks disparagingly about her ex-husband it often has a convoluted effect; the child may well side with the parent who's gone.

A patient once told me that whenever she was sick her divorced mother pointedly told her that her father wouldn't visit her. The tone implied something weightier than a missed visit. When she needed glasses, her mother reminded her that her father wasn't around to take her for a fitting. That tone again. When she was in a play, her father wouldn't attend. "How was I supposed to feel?" she asked. "Everything was said in a tone that meant he didn't love me at all or that I should appreciate what a burden she had in raising me alone. As I grew older, I thought, what poor judgment you must have had, Mother, to have chosen a man who never cared about his family. She could never understand why I'd think that."

Single parents may hold a child too closely out of emotional need. They require reassurance that a spouse may have indeed left, but the child still needs and loves them, and doesn't hold them entirely responsible for the dissolution of the marriage. Going it alone as a single parent is difficult, and women should be careful that their distress doesn't get in a child's way too much. A child needs both parents, and if an ex-husband is available, don't let bitterness disturb whatever communication the child may have with him.

# On Being Alone

"I'm alone . . . I'm all alone." Women say these words and their skins prickle, their hearts palpitate, tears flow. Those who cannot do without a man are happy for any masculine company. Fearful that they may never again meet a kindred soul, they rush into a relationship that either duplicates their failed marriage or is completely wrong for them, and they are soon up against the same old fear—being alone.

Rather than go through the rigors of the adjustment period without her first husband, Loretta opted to marry after six months alone. She had panicked as she went through a number of phases she didn't understand. Feeling hurt and abandoned, enraged that she wasn't loved or appreciated by a man, Loretta, like many divorcées, first became promiscuous. She yearned for attention, the physical comfort of a warm body. Following this came a period of testing out other people—a sudden fierceness or brutal honesty directed at others. She needed to feel strong, on top of things. She then began to frantically look for another mate, venturing into singles bars, joining clubs for single parents, visiting resorts. This left her feeling breathless, disappointed and disinclined to go out. Then she met John.

John was twenty-four and ready to settle down; Loretta was thirty-one. "When I first got divorced," she said, "I was all right, considering myself on a new adventure. That quickly wore off. I needed stability, and my young son needed continuity, since my ex-husband not only moved out but relocated to Europe.

"When John first proposed to me, I thought it was ridiculous—he was basically a boy; I was an older woman with a child. But something in me snapped. I began to feel myself turning into my own mother. My father died when I was two years old and my mother never recovered from his death—she was haunted her entire life by the loss. Sometimes she'd wish me and my sister were out of her life so she'd have a better chance to attract a man. On those bleak days, she felt we were in her way, preventing her happiness and a traditional married life." (Thirty years ago it was unusual for a young widow or divorcée to remarry—especially if she had children.)

"So I did the unthinkable—I said yes and I practically begged John to marry me. A friend of mine always says, 'As it begins, so will it end,' and I wish I'd paid attention to her. This is what happened on my wedding day: John refused to have a party, after a marriage at city hall. Nor could I invite friends over for a drink. He wanted to marry me to have me, but he felt that if he showed *how much,* he wouldn't be manly. To him, celebrating a wedding day was admitting weakness! He enjoyed my son before we married, but that soon changed when he became a stepfather. He was never again sympathetic to Charlie and went for weeks without speaking to him."

Loretta found herself a man, but not a companion. John wasn't ready for marriage and neither was Loretta. Both needed to establish the solidity and comfort of family life, but chose each other for all the wrong reasons. She was still alone within her marriage; so was he.

Their marriage lasted nine years, but it wasn't all gloom, isolation and quarrels. "John was an interesting man in his way," Loretta added. "He believed creativity deserved attention." Loretta had a talent for designing, and John encouraged her to try her hand at fabric design. "He more or less pushed me into a profession. Ironically, it was easier to phase out my marriage because I had a job two years before I knew we'd eventually break up. An abrupt separation would have been too terrifying for me and my son. A little success at work eventually helped build my confidence to where I just asked him to leave."

Loretta missed John terribly when he left, but the miracle was feeling that she'd "come back to herself." In both her marriages, she'd viewed the union as a solemn process—two people embarking on an eternal life together—rather than as an adventure in communication and affection. "If I've learned anything from both marriages," she concluded, "it's what I'd want next—a deep friendship, compassion and a compatible sexual partner. I look forward to finding it."

Relearning the single life is hard on the nervous system. You wonder if you can build friendships with men and just relax. You wonder if you are destined to continue the hunt for a mate until you're too old to try. There is no guarantee that you'll find a man. There's no guarantee that if you do, he'll be inclined to make your life and his better. The only guarantee you have is the measure of your own self-worth. If you keep measuring yourself as the rejectee, as the sad soul life left behind to never find another man, you can never accept the fact that you're worthy of a good life of your own making.

"To embark on new and more effective ways of relating and loving is to rock the boat of who you think you may be," says Mel Krantzler in *Learning to Love Again*. "Of course, you can settle for much less in life by not rocking that boat. Ahead lies the enormous positive reward for which the risk of seeing yourself in a new light will be taken. Behind you lies the familiar, comfortable discomfort of knowing that nothing new will happen in your life and therefore a meaningful love relationship is a hopeless dream."

We both aver that the choice is up to you.

"To rock the boat" means you can relinquish pain and are clear to love again, to *learn* to love again, if you must. Steeped in bitterness, no man, no matter how accomplished and giving, will look acceptable to you. To rock the boat in your life so you can be happier requires an understanding of your skills beyond the home front. Divorce may have proven to you that you won't always have a man to support you. On the average—and this is shocking—after a divorce, a woman's standard of living, with her children, drops 73 percent, while a divorced man's increases 42 percent!

If you are married and do not work, take this time to consider some difficult and painful questions: *What would you do if you were suddenly alone?* How would you meet that challenge? Can you take a note pad and pencil and write down where the family money is now? Do you know exactly where to find your assets? Whose name are they in? Could you get a job if necessary or train for a better one?

The following might be the test of your strength and courage if you're just starting out in the job market: Are you willing to take a low-level job when you return to the work force, knowing you can advance or move to another position once you are trained? Now's the time, while you are still in your marriage, to see how an outside job suits you. You will discover what it takes to get up at seven in the morning, deal with chores, the kids, and get to work by nine, do a job, come home, make dinner and do whatever else needs tending to in the evenings.

The bitter truth is that a good many women wind up spending a portion of their lives alone because of death, divorce or desertion. Thrust out into the world, many falter, become emotionally enfeebled, lazy, too immersed in bitterness to grow . . . and grow up! *The way to stay insecure about your ability to accomplish anything is by doing nothing*. The more we keep ourselves in the same place, the more leaks will spring in the boat that wasn't rocked.

# Getting Better While You're Still Married

This is a simple exercise, one that could greatly assist you in clarifying what your marriage means to you and how to improve it while you can. A big order, but you can do it. Three types of women will most benefit from it:

- Women who have become disoriented in their marriages because all the control has passed into their husbands' hands
- Women who have found conflicts over power, control and dominance becoming daily battlefields
- Newlyweds

You will need your husband's cooperation for this exercise. Let him know how much this means to you. This is your marriage: save it!

Now the exercise: Pick a day—if you're sentimental, let it be your anniversary—and clear everything out of sight. Let there be no distractions in the background so each of you can interrupt with comments. Stick to the subject. Concentrate. Sit down with your husband, give him a sheet of paper, take one for yourself and start with this list: Write down five qualities you like about your spouse; ask him to do the same for you. Write down five qualities that irritate you and that you'd like to see changed; he should do the same about you. Now exchange papers.

Try not to be angry or hurt when you see the list of qualities he thinks need changing. Instead of denying you have these attributes, or defending them, listen to what he has to say. Are you too quick-tempered and impatient? Acknowledge it if it's true. Think about it. Can you remember quarrels starting because you were on edge and spoke a little too sharply to your husband and children? For his part, can he acknowledge that he thinks it funny to belittle you in the company of his friends? Can he see that it hurts you and makes him look less of a man, not more? Do you defer to him in all decision making? Does he always veto your suggestions?

Now pick one quality that needs improving and work on it. Keep it conscious; allow him to point out when you slip back into old patterns. Do the same for him. Finally, set up a number of *mutual* goals you'd like to accomplish over the next year. Talk them out; be sure they are realistic goals, ones that will improve the relationship and how you live. Put these notes in a plastic binder where you keep the family pictures. In one year, or six months, if you're diligent, take out the notes and see what progress you've made.

This is a serious exercise because it will give you a sure and accurate chronicle of how you work as a team. You will be able to observe how much cooperation there is between you in decision making, how you spend time together, how you honor each other's promises and needs. You will see how committed you are to changing! These lists can help you deal effectively with jealousies, inadequacies, fears, power struggles, demonstrations of affection and trust—all by what progress and effort both of you put into making the marriage work.

My husband and I began our marriage nearly thirty years ago with the $300 I'd saved from a summer job. For many years, a double-dipped ice cream cone for two was a luxury. But we've worked hard and are comfortable now. What matters most to me is that we've basically helped each other grow, enhanced each other's lives. We've had unpleasant times and struck out at each other, but we've also had good times. I've known Stephen since I was fourteen years old, when I discovered him at the beach in Brooklyn, working on a perfect tan. Over the years, we've come to the point at which if we ever decide to leave each other, it would be with a compassionate goodbye. Not less. I would hope that there'd be the knowledge that the other has changed, and that parting would not diminish what we have shared during three decades. I would hope that we would ask of each other no punishments, no bitterness. Just a fair and friendly parting. And that it was a great journey, but it ended.

# 7

## Start the Crisis Without Me

"Say yes to everything until someone says, 'Have you had enough?'" These are words from the remarkable Patricia Hill Burnett, portrait painter and activist, speaking about possibilities—the exploration of life. She is now in her early sixties, vivid, involved, fulfilled creatively by her work and the work she does for others. Patricia exemplifies how a woman can transform her life through work.

Her parents divorced when she was three years old, and she was raised by a working mother—an unusual situation for the mid-1920s. Her artistic talent showed itself early and she was encouraged, given painting lessons. But it didn't occur to her in her early years that painting could be her life's work. While she was in college, Patricia modeled, and on a lark, auditioned for the female lead in the classic radio show "The Green Hornet." She got the part although she wasn't yet twenty. About that time, her mother remarried, with Patricia's enthusiastic encouragement. "My mother's gynecologist had fallen in love with her, but after nearly twenty years of being divorced, she was still hesitant about remarrying. I went to her and insisted—got her to say yes. I thought he'd be the most wonderful husband to her and father to me. They were married for forty years, until he died last year at the age of ninety-nine."

When they first met, her stepfather's son dared Patricia to enter a beauty pageant. Patricia thought winning had little to do with real beauty and talent and more to do with how a woman presented herself. All three qualities were in her favor—she was crowned Miss Michigan. This made her eligible for the Miss America pageant. In that contest, she was first runner-up. The title gave her the opportunity for a Hollywood screen test, but as she reports, "I wasn't an actress, but I wasn't hungry enough or motivated enough to go for it." Patricia returned to Michigan.

She married a doctor when she was twenty-four and got pregnant—but the marriage didn't last. Three years later, she married again, to a strong, successful man. With him she had three more children and a comfortable enough life, but had a deep sense of longing to paint again. For nearly twenty years she was the dutiful wife, deferring to her husband, living according to his directives. But she needed something more—something for herself. She began timidly sketching at the kitchen table, delighted when people would sit for her. It was a beginning. Then, when she was in her forties, she took the big step and moved her easel and paints into a studio. She began to receive commissions for portraits, and, with her talent, she soon became well known.

In 1969, she felt a restlessness, frustration with her relationship with her husband, the conflicts that were arising from being the "good" wife and having a career. "I began speaking to other women, discussing the problems we were facing at home. All of us needed a support group. With a friend, I convened all the professional women we could think of in Detroit, and by the end of the meeting, we'd all become a part of what would be one of the more powerful chapters of NOW." Patricia was elected president of this branch of the National Organization of Women, a post she held for two years before moving to the international board.

"Feminism transformed me in a number of important ways," she said. "For so many years, all my anger was directed at my husband. I believed he was preventing me from being what I could be. I realized it wasn't up to him to give me permission to go out and paint or work for a cause, it was up to me. He was a strong, traditional man, formed by a family with very traditional ideas about a woman's role—and that was to stay at home. This is what he'd always wanted in me.

"I didn't know what it was to disobey," she continued. "I'd obeyed my mother, then a forceful husband. What I finally did was change my attitude toward my husband and recognize who he was. I found myself falling in love with him again after so many years of resenting his power over me. If anything kept us together during those years before he died, it was an acceptance of him and what I needed to do for myself."

Then she added this thought: "If women learn to care for themselves and care for each other—and not be so judgmental—the world can open up. It allows you to experience the joys of life—even the joys of growing older."

"Nobody is going to save you; that's your job. Save yourself. If you don't like where you are, get out of there. The object is not for them to like you, the object is for them to listen to you. Nobody knows what you want except you. And nobody will be as sorry as you if you don't get it," wrote playwright Marsha Norman in the *New York Times,* describing "the sermons" the late Lillian Hellman "delivered so freely." There's more.

"Your family thinks of you as a pet, you have to leave them. They are just where you came from, they are not what you are. They will give you everything they have, but that will not make you want it or know what to do with it. Wanting some other way to live is proof enough of deserving it. Having it is hard work, but not having it is sheer hell."

Wise words. Wonderful words.

Traditionally, women have been closely acquainted with the "sheer hell" of not having. The more patient of us are also good at waiting for others to share their bounties with us. This is *getting,* then, not having through one's own efforts—that glorious feeling that comes with self-generated, self-motivated, creative *having.* And as with Patti, it will be up to you to get it through productive work.

Women once considered employment a sign of failure—they "had to" work because their husbands didn't earn enough, or they weren't "lucky" enough to have a husband. If they did work, there were only a few acceptable occupations open to them—teaching, secretarial, clerical or nursing jobs. In that more conservative climate, if a woman worked, it was thought to be harmful to the health of her family. Thus, before the 1970s there weren't many "latchkey children"—the progeny of working mothers, each carrying a house key on a string around their neck because Mom wasn't there when they came home from school. I was one of them for a number of my formative years. My mother was frustrated by having to work; or, at least, it was *expected* that she would find the condition frustrating, not enriching.

Work is no longer a sadness in the family, proof that we selected a man who couldn't provide for his own without assistance from the woman he was supposed to support. Women once apologized for their jobs, belittled them, diminished their importance in their lives. But when a child of a working mother—rather a *son* of a working mother—was successful, Mom was revered for the sacrifices she made for him. While she worked, it was a burden—her lot. The true blessing, we'd been taught, was to give ourselves up to the marriage—to be provided for. Ideally, the good life was to be pampered by marrying well—a guarantee of freedom from obligations, drudgery, subways, cramped offices, standing on one's feet eight hours a day. Work, then, had no payoff but a paycheck.

It's not news that since the mid-1960s women have broken out and are being employed in fields that were once male enclaves. The working woman is no longer an anomaly, a flamingo that has wandered into a flock of geese. But she is still suspect, especially if she distinguishes herself by showing ambition. In general, it is okay to be a movie star, but if you produce the movie it is not okay. Or it's okay to be an executive secretary, not a corporation president.

Women and work and women and ambition still are not easily blended combinations because women and men both protect outmoded tradition. "It's women like you who make life difficult for me," many women remind me, angry about those of us who go out into the world and try to make changes, accomplish something for ourselves and others. May those for whom I make life difficult never need to test their ability to survive when they are hit by an unfamiliar or threatening situation—death, divorce or desertion of a spouse. May those for whom work is a crisis always have a cushion. May those who do not even work on a volunteer basis and are content to minister to family and friends have a pleasant life. The rest of us need *productive* work whether we are single, married, divorced, widowed.

Let's examine some facts.

By the year 2000 it is predicted that the rising divorce rate will mean more serial marriages. By 1990, almost 50 percent of all children will have experienced the effects of divorce. Economic conditions will require more single and married women in the work force. Increasing longevity among women will give them an average of seven more years without a partner. Women will marry later, opting for more experience in business and the professions. By the turn of the century, two-thirds of all American wives and most single female parents will hold jobs. Girls as well as boys will be trained to be providers instead of being reared to relate only to the functioning of the home. Housework will be an equal opportunity job.

The nature of opportunities in work is changing for us. Ten years ago, the nation's space program did not recruit women to train them as astronauts. Now there are eight. A decade ago, the largest banks in the United States resisted promoting women to vice-presidential positions; now there are nearly one hundred. In 1972, women were appointed to one management job in eight within companies citing one hundred or more employees. Now the figures are one in five. Ten years ago, thirteen women served in the House of Representatives. As of January 1984, a record twenty-one women serve there, while two hold Senate seats. Nine hundred women are in state legislatures as compared to three hundred ten years ago. And in July of 1984, one feisty

Congresswoman from Queens, New York, made headlines and history by taking her place as the first woman vice-presidential candidate on the Democratic ticket.

Sound impressive? Progressive? Are advances as exceptional as they appear? Here's the flip side of the figures. Only 5 percent of executives in top corporations are women; 10 percent of the astronauts are women, 12 percent of state legislators are women, and 2 percent of United States Senators are women.

All of us, achievers and doubters, share a history about work. The picture looks like this: Historically, women were neither encouraged nor permitted much leeway to achieve in business—excellence beyond the secretarial pool was none too "nice." Reasons for this go beyond the separation of the duties of motherhood and tending families (the "feminine" position) from fulfilling work (the "masculine" principle). *Men don't want to share power.* Once you know this, you can correct your strategies for dealing with the inequities in this contrary world. Anthony Astrachan, writing in *Ms.*, lets us in on how men feel about power. In describing why women confront male anger or negative feedback in the workplace, he tells us it's "something men seldom talk about—the question of power. When women go to work, men feel a loss of power and what sociologist William J. Goode calls 'a loss of centrality, a decline in the extent to which they are the center of attention.'"

So, Astrachan avers, men may love their wives, daughters, mothers, feel proud of their accomplishments and happy for the money these women bring home. But here's the rub: "At home, those positive emotions help to balance our basic fear of female power—the power to give birth, and the power of the mother we knew as babies. At work, we are frightened when we see a woman peer combine those powers with the power of work, the power to reshape the external world, and we resist change more strongly."

Many of us needed work and discovered it was work that satisfied us more than the homemaker's role. And we were not content to toil at low-level jobs until retirement. Few of us knew how to achieve; we just knew how to aspire. As more of us poured into the world of business, we learned quickly by watching the men above us—and the few women who had struggled through to success. Instruction was pretty thorough— we learned how to play ball with the boys, what constituted a success strategy, which outfit sold us as promotable, when to talk ourselves into jobs for which we were in no way qualified, how to decorate the office, where to sit at meetings so others knew if we were top dog or run of the litter. Women observed men at the game of business, learned the tricks, and in many cases applied them.

Not all women will rise to top jobs no matter how much coaching they get—and that's okay. For many, work is important in itself, not just because it brings tangible rewards. Rewards are *not* the point; productive work *is*—and it is productive and worthwhile work only if you judge it so. Being involved in work prepares you for any eventuality. It is part of a growth process that helps you take care of yourself. If you surrender your care to someone else, you may find yourself at his mercy.

An example comes to mind. This story aptly describes a woman's vulnerabilities in marriage—and what can happen when productive work is given up for the illusion of productive love.

Debbie's story is an extreme statement about surrender and its consequences—I do not in any way believe that all married women face such punishment. I offer this case as a cautionary tale, to show you how relationships can get out of control and *be* controlling unless you have something that's your own.

Debbie came for a consultation with me when she was twenty-nine years old and separated from her husband about two weeks. "I have no feelings," she murmured in desolate tones. "My life is over." What had happened to her?

Debbie had been enrolled in her first year of dental school when she met Don, a man with two more years of law school ahead of him. Don was getting some financial help from his parents for tuition, but when he and Debbie decided to marry, Debbie dropped out of school and got a job in a dentist's office to support them. Don promised that when he was set up in practice, he'd put her through school.

About six months into the marriage, Don suggested that since Debbie was still sexually "immature," she needed a number of lovers to "awaken" her. These lovers, Don continued, would be of his choosing, men he knew from school, friends, whoever struck his fancy. The final stipulation was that he would charge them a small fee. There'd be an extra bonus then to her "development"—cash they needed. Debbie resisted. Don was furious. Then she agreed, unable to tolerate his displeasure. She loved him, she thought, what choice did she have? He had this *power* over her.

When Don graduated from law school, he joined forces with two friends and opened an office. He and Debbie moved into a sprawling suburban house. Debbie, always compliant, said nothing when Don put the house in his name only. Don bought a top-of-the-line Porsche—*his* car—while Debbie was stranded without one. Don reminded her that there wasn't enough money for two: she'd have to rely on him to take her wherever she needed to go. Since he'd already convinced her to quit her job and work at his office for minimal pay, he saw no reason for her to waste money on another car.

When they were married for eight years, Don announced coolly, "I've just called my parents to tell them we're getting a divorce. I want you to leave." Debbie had believed that her marriage would last forever: how could it end? She had meekly followed Don's rules; wasn't she more than amply a "good wife"? Hadn't she done her best to make the marriage a happy one? She'd prostituted herself, given up a career goal, worked for him for nearly no pay, committed herself to his success, and now he wanted her out. When she asked him how and with what she was to leave, Don offhandedly suggested she hock her diamond wedding band.

"I'd never felt such panic," Debbie told me. "I had no money, no place to go, and my husband was kicking me out. Why? I still don't know why. I asked him if he didn't feel some sense of responsibility toward me—I'd given him everything he wanted. He said I was old enough to take care of myself."

Debbie's slavish devotion to Don did not pay off as she had hoped it would. She believed that if she pleased him, the time would come when he would please her. He would not only share his success to support her through dental school, but their marriage would be perfect. Debbie did not heed the true messages behind what Don had in mind. First, he told her that she wasn't sexually satisfying to him, that she needed "experience." Second, that she was, in effect, worthless as a person but worth something when her lovers paid for her. Finally, Debbie's work and goals were not important to him; therefore, by his reasoning, they could not be important to her. Debbie's commitment was to him alone, and that would take precedence over anything else in her life. After eight years of marriage, she was emotionally and financially dependent on him. She had more, in every way, the day she married Don than the day she left, eight years later.

If any case argues for a woman caring for herself, protecting herself within a marriage, it is Debbie's. Hers is a particularly dramatic example, yet many women's lives parallel it one way or another. To be a caretaker; the selfless support system to a man; the too passive, acquiescent wife who has no power at all over her life is to be in a very high-risk profession. Try to remember that while there are benefits to being a caretaker, there are also penalties. You have no guarantee that a man will always be there. But *you* are always there for you.

What about Debbie? Where can she start? She's thirty years old now, with some fifty years of life ahead of her, barring unforeseen catastrophe. Time is in her favor. She's alive, bright, sensitive, and though she may not know it, capable of making enormous changes. She has lived as a man's possession within his marriage (not *their* marriage), allowed herself to be vulnerable and hurt, but her plea for help indicates that she still has hope. She must reach a point where she can give herself permission to grow. It may be frightening for her, but living within Don's life, where she was nothing, was much more so. And to become something? She will start her journey, as many women have, exploring what she can do to enrich herself inside and outside marriage.

Is it possible to turn a life around?

# The 180-Degree Turnabout

Men who've switched careers midstream are no longer anomalies. In the past, they stayed with one kind of work for life, not even switching companies often. Today, that's changed. A doctor takes down his shingle at the age of fifty and turns to photography. Forty-year-old bankers donate their pin-stripe suits to the Salvation Army and spend the remainder of their lives plowing the north forty in some remote area—farming appeals to them. A thirty-eight-year-old steelworker goes to school and becomes a computer specialist. Midlife does not mean the beginning of the end to these men with dreams. They have only so much time on this earth, and commit themselves to spending it in the manner that matters most to them.

Career changes are no longer remarkable for men—or for women. One reason is that we've become a less constricted society. We no longer believe that a person, male or female, is obliged to select a career in his or her late teens and stick to it until retirement or death. Now we can explore options, develop a new skill that will take us to a totally unrelated field, while still working at a long- or short-term job. Or we can pick up where we left off ten, twenty or thirty years before and start again. This is the 180-degree turnabout, and it can work miracles when there's a lot of commitment to yourself.

Where does the turnabout start? Perhaps you're a woman like Debbie, who gave up a career to help her husband attain his goals. If you are still interested in that career, whether it's dentistry, dressmaking or working as a travel agent, investigate every aspect of what you need to do to achieve your goal. Start somewhere. And the woman who's worked part time over the years while tending her home and children? The turnabout may come when she decides to enter the work force full time at a career that will demand more time away from home. The dedicated housewife experiencing "burnout" may well know it's time to seek gratification in fulfilling work outside the home. The careerist, dissatisfied with her choice, may, as with her male counterpart, jump from one field to another— from law to textile design, or from working as an executive secretary to running a flower shop.

When you actually get out there and change your life around with fulfilling work, you may not start out at a top pay scale, but you will be out there, part of the world and moving up if you so choose. By using your personal power, you will be projected along your course, meeting challenges and making your life count.

The 180-degree turnabout requires that you make decisions that will be in your best interest. That means choosing work that can take you from square one to square two. It will allow you to hone skills, learn how to talk to people in meetings or on the phone, discover your strengths and weaknesses. Some women, just starting out, feel somewhat inadequate, though in truth they are not. They choose work that interests them, but are sometimes at a loss to use their abilities in their best interests. Betty's story is an example.

Betty is a housewife with abundant energy and three children in school. She applies her organizational skills, enthusiasm and sense of commitment to working countless hours as president of a soap star's fan club. This is wonderful for the star, but not as wonderful for Betty as she had originally thought. Here is a woman who has all the qualities to be successful in business or charitable work, a woman who should be paid for her efforts or at least receive more than an occasional thank you. But she is timid about getting a job, competing "out there." Working gratis for the star gives her a way out, keeps her, basically, an adoring woman, not an effective one. She is treading water.

It's easy to fall into jobs where there's little tangible return for the energy and time you put in. If you do not need the money paid you for the work, selective time (as with someone like Betty) can be spent on the less glamorous in life who need commitment and devotion. Money may not be the reward, but that connection to others less fortunate than you is priceless. You are appreciated, challenged, spiritually enriched.

If you do need the money, volunteer work offers a multitude of possibilities for developing skills that can be listed on your résumé when you seek a job. For example, few businesses would turn down a woman with experience in organizing projects, doing mailings, putting out newsletters or bulletins, or counseling others.

## Growing Up with Work

Turning thirty is a milestone in more ways than one. For too many of us, the period after three decades of life seems like the start of a downhill race. We expect to hit the end of the slope in a few seconds flat, fatalities in time's little game. We dread thirty because it signals the onset of aging—lost youth, loss of opportunities, unthinkable loneliness. We wonder, "Where has it all gone?"

Fatalistic thinking like this is not only outdated but

counterproductive. At thirty your image in a mirror may not reflect the way you looked at eighteen, but why would you want it to? You have lived. And what lies ahead is not a disquieting onset of woes, but a shift into true adolescence.

I'll give that to you again. At thirty, you may begin to build toward a new adolescence. Chalk up the years behind you as a well-spent childhood in which you were impulsive, irreverent, defiant, temperamental, skeptical. You were catching on to who you are. By thirty, you can establish who you are and what you want. You can finally cooperate with yourself to achieve your goals. The upcoming decade between thirty and forty encompasses your real adolescence, and you can experiment, accept that you are not doomed to another forty years of the same, by changing into a smart cookie. This new adolescence allows you to begin a reappraisal of your roles; to stage new challenges and meet them. If they turn into battles, you will discover how to emerge from them with only a few scratches, maybe a scar or two, but it won't be shell shock that'll get you. The real danger is in not fighting to get what's right for you. Know that a few quick-to-heal bruises along the way do not mean defeat.

Let me repeat Freud's assertion that the foundation for the good life rests on productive love and productive work. Until recently, women, who constitute over half of the American population, thought Freud was speaking only of men, because our assumption, as women, was that we had to carve out a life exclusively from productive love. Productive love was our lodestar, even if the road was rutted, rocky, or impassable. With little else to sustain us, we shambled on.

I do not mean to imply that we should give up productive love—motherhood, family life, husbands, ties to children. Not at all. I don't think that every young mother should necessarily work: it's delightful to feel good about staying home with small children during those wonderful years until they are of school age. These are important years for laying down basic values for your children, establishing closeness and giving them a sense of security. I *am* appealing to you to take the next step: *Let go of that need to tend others to the exclusion of your own development.* Tackle the reality of your own life. At some point those children you dote on will fight for their right to become individuals, to detach themselves from you. This separation is critical for their development, but you will be left at home. Studies show that the average woman spends about an hour and a half a day cleaning her house. What will she do with the rest of the time? What will she do *in addition to* being a homemaker?

If you want to live the good life, bend Freud's dictum: With productive love *and* productive work you can make love more productive and produce something for yourself and others. Work allows you more chances to grow; to stretch yourself. It enables you to meet new people, to explore challenges, even to experience the pain of rejection or initial failure. These experiences make you stronger. With work you can learn to cope with difficult situations, to not take yourself too seriously, and to not take criticism as if the earth were opening under your feet. Work teaches you to shrug off uncomplimentary or hurtful remarks, to think, maturely, "He's had a bad day," rather than muttering angrily as you contemplate the snub, insult, or inattentiveness. But when your home alone circumscribes your world, your husband is an extension of you; in fact, the greater part of you. Every time he insists he cannot do something for you, it strikes you that he is being deliberately irresponsible in adding to your burdens. And if your children say no, you perceive them as deliberately not showing respect—they are ingrates, selfish, spoiled. They are the center of your universe.

Productive work, by contrast, provides perspective on life. No longer isolated in an insulated haven, you needn't search for busywork like relining the kitchen shelves. Productive work is what you think is worthwhile at the moment, but it also offers you the opportunity to take care of yourself after that moment is over. Studies show that women who work may initially take jobs because they need the income to help get family finances above water. But, surprise! Money is not the prime benefit. The prime benefit is self-esteem. And these studies include women with many different kinds of jobs—factory workers, retail store employees, bank tellers, corporate executives.

There are women who devote their lives to rearing their children, decorating the house, perfecting a tennis backstroke, planting an herb garden and planning dinner parties. If that's agreeable to both a woman and her husband, wonderful. But what if he dies? What if he leaves her for another woman? What if he becomes ill and can't work? And the big question: What if he needs her to rally her forces and get out there and contribute? How will she take care of herself, of *him,* if a drop in his earning power changes her lifestyle dramatically? I worry about these women, whose numbers grow yearly. These are the women who've had the privilege of security for most of their lives, but may not be able to adapt to a crisis.

With productive work you have the potential to create in yourself a better human being. You can be kinder, more competent, more able to see the world from another's perspective. With productive work comes maturity. It may not make you the best negotiator or boss, but it makes you a more resilient person.

If you sit back without making an effort and wait for a job, for a man, for a life to fall into your lap, you may spend time on this earth regretting that you didn't take a step. No action, no results.

*The best insurance policy any woman has is a marketable skill.* Our mothers used to preach about the value of a teaching certificate or familiarity with a typewriter. They told us that secretarial work or teaching could be valuable skills for us to fall back on. This is still true. If you validate your teaching certificate yearly, putting in the required number of days in school, you have a cushion. A little practice at the keyboard gets the secretary back to her old speed.

# Excuses, Excuses . . .

Even with all these good reasons to look for productive work, many women are intimidated by the prospect. They resort to a series of classic, well-defined excuses that keep them tied to home or self-defeating situations. Let's take a look at a few of these excuses in the hope that exploring and understanding them will help you overcome them.

## THE PAY'S LOUSY AND SO IS THE BOSS

One agonizing situation I see regularly in my practice is that of a woman anywhere in age from the mid-thirties to the early sixties who has been abandoned and is suddenly confronted by harsh economic necessity. Now that her husband is gone, she has no choice but to work, but she often knows little about the intricacies of the workplace. Suddenly she's forced to face the painful fact that at her level of skills, she may be capable of earning only the minimum wage or a few dollars above it. Humiliated by the lilliputian pay scale offered for her services, feeling demeaned that she has to work after a lifetime of being taken care of, she gives up.

Or, smart (or desperate) enough to take a job at starting pay, thinking she can advance, get experience and move on, she is soon intimidated by those who supervise her day—a woman her daughter's age, or worse, her own age. Today, the boss in a blue gabardine suit is as likely to be a woman as a man. The excuse maker can never work for a suitable enough boss. She is frightened by younger women or women her own age who remind her that once, in the far distant and glorious past, someone made it possible for her to be protected in her nest. She struggles to speak the same language as her boss. If she can't, she'll seek a translator who'll tell her what she wants to hear—an ally as steeped in resentment as she is. If her boss is male and young, she may resent him for having authority over her; he's her "son." An older man reminds her of what she's missing—a protector. There's a temptation, though, to pamper the "son" and flirtatiously "scold" the older man. And if either man resists her tending and requests a more sober, professional demeanor, she is hurt.

An older woman can go through a painful period of adjustment as she is directed through the workday by a younger person whom she believes ought to be working for *her*, by dint of age alone. When jealousy or misunderstanding exists between her and her boss, an older woman feels especially sensitive. Janice La-

Rouche and Regina Ryan offer advice for this woman in *Strategies for Women at Work:* "Women tend to make moral judgments from a frame of reference that blocks their understanding of movement in the workplace. They judge workplace practices using family and friendship values, putting human needs above all." They must learn new insights about relations in the work setting, the authors continue, "*how* the system works, and *why* it works the way it does. It is not enough to stand aside and judge it."

If you don't like the pay scale or who's running the store, you may lose by heading for the exit. Pay scales go up and so can aspirations. Put in that first year of getting adjusted to the work world. Think about how to make the job a better one, and learn office politics. Brooding about what cannot be changed will forever hold you back if you let it.

## IF I DO SOMETHING FOR MYSELF, MY HUSBAND WILL PUNISH ME

This is the worst form of misguided theorizing, for alarmist thinking never got anyone out of the house. There's an old joke about the middle-aged mother who hadn't bathed in years—she feared her son would call while she was in the tub and she wouldn't hear the phone. A silly joke perhaps, but a good number of women apply similar reasoning, if not to bathing then to other aspects of their lives. With grown children out of the house and fully entrenched in their own lives, Mother stays home *in case*. The fantasy of being needed by her children on a twenty-four-hour basis is immobilizing. Where can she go? Where does she dare go? What if she's not on call—will her children perish?

And what if she's over the hurdle of keeping herself

available to her children at a moment's notice? It is now her husband who likes her at home, who demands that she be there, doing nothing but chatting with neighbors and taking care of his territory. This husband may or may not arrive home promptly for dinner at six. He may or may not have much to say to her when he's around, yet he's comforted by knowing he's in command. Because he keeps her in her place, she is powerless to find her own place in the world.

This problem is not limited to older women: younger women are also beset by it. The case of the threatened spouse is common. Helen is one such victim. Born into privilege, she married young and quickly had two children. Helen was raised to be the quintessential "good girl." Her brother got all the support toward a career; Helen was advised to marry well and as young as she could. What else could she do? Right out of high school she married Rob, a man five years her senior, an up-and-coming executive in a major corporation.

Helen lacked for nothing. By twenty-one, she had two children; by twenty-four she was beginning to search for fulfillment in other ways—she wanted to go back to school, get a degree. Rob forbade it. Forcefully, he told her she didn't need an education—he would take care of her. Helen insisted it was important for her to have something of her own other than just watching the children. Rob became abusive, telling her she was dumb, incapable of concentrating on anything requiring more than minimal attention. She enrolled in school anyway.

Helen's marriage was suffering on a number of levels then—Rob's cruelty increased: he was teaching the children to be equally abusive toward her. He flaunted his extramarital affairs, humiliating Helen. "I wanted to leave him after a few years, but I stayed because I was afraid to be alone," she told me. "Then I worried, eventually, about how it would affect the kids. Finally it got to me and I asked for a divorce. To my surprise, Rob got married eight weeks after our divorce came through—he married the latest of his girlfriends while we'd been married." Helen and Rob agreed to joint custody of their children.

Helen went it alone, continuing to attend school while she adjusted to single life. Two years later, she met another man and married him. "Ed is a kind, supportive, wonderful man," she said. "Not punishing like my first husband was. And though he's proud of me and encourages me, I worry that if I continue in school, something will happen to this marriage too. But Ed assures me that he won't turn on me like Rob did."

The only thorn in Helen's life is her first husband's influence on her children. "He wants them to live with him, and so makes me the bad guy. I'm the woman who dared defy him. I'm the mother who dared go back to school a few hours a day while they were in school. He tells them that I don't care about them, that I'm selfish for wanting a career. Things are touchy now between me and the children because of Rob, but I feel that when they're older, they'll be more able to judge for themselves and truly know I love them."

## MY HUSBAND WILL TAKE CARE OF ME

Nothing sounds sweeter than to hear a man tell you not to worry about money, especially when the money he brings home is substantial. Here's a fur coat, new living room furniture, a trip to Martinique. He works hard; he's ambitious enough; he's responsible for you.

We all are a little afraid of growing older, but

we're also afraid of growing up. We want that cushion, and the longer we've had it, the more we need it. First we were protected from life by parents, then by a husband who took over. There is the illusion of being totally protected by a man, the insulation of external trappings. But it *is* an illusion. He may not always be there. And, most of all, money is no reason not to work. Gloria Vanderbilt works; Jacqueline Onassis works. Both need productive work. Money may be insulating, but it's no excuse not to grow.

## What You Can Do

Work is as creative a process in its way as giving birth. Instead of birthing children, you will give birth to ideas and a new sense of self. This new adolescence is a generative time, an opportunity to carve out a place for yourself outside the home. Within your renaissance during those years from forty to fifty, you can make real choices about where your life is going. You will be on the way to maturity and entitlement. Let's bring you closer to action.

The woman reading these pages who's never worked wants to know how to get started. Or the single woman might be stuck in a dead-end job, not knowing where she can go next. The older married woman just on the brink of joining the work force asks the same question: Who am I really? What do I like to do? Where do I fit in? How do I get employed?

There are countless ways to enter the job market. The traditional routes are well known—answering classified ads, going to employment agencies, keeping your ears open for leads. Women who've decided on a job that requires advanced education enroll in technical or academic courses. Social work, special education, psychology—these are a few of the choices open to women who are comfortable with careers in the helping professions. Others prefer industry and take courses in computer technology, financial management, administration, real estate sales—these are women who are more at ease in high-pressure, money-producing fields.

When you need assistance in sorting out what you want to do, ask for it! There are tests available at career-counseling agencies and business schools that can clarify what direction to take. One such test, the Strong-Campbell Interest Inventory, helps pinpoint how you feel about a number of areas. It could help you select work that you will like. For example, it could help you decide whether you should work in a large organization or if you are a self-starter who works efficiently and productively on her own. You will see if you prefer continually changing activities or not; if you like competitive activities or more contemplative work. These tests are useful because they ask questions about preferences and tastes that you may have overlooked. A number of books can offer counseling too: *Women Working Home: The Homebased Business Guide and Directory*, by Marion Behr and Wendy Lazar (WWH Press); *What Color Is Your Parachute?*, by Richard Bolles (Ten Speed Press); *Jobs of the Future: The Five Hundred Best Jobs—Where They'll Be and How to Get Them*, by Marvin Cetron and Marcia Appel (McGraw-Hill); and *Janice LaRouche's Strategies for Women at Work*, by Janice LaRouche and Regina Ryan (Avon).

Sometimes a professional opportunity arises when you least expect it. A number of women who have been in therapy with me have discovered that being both action-oriented and introspective can be combined in a helping profession. They like giving others a supporting hand. What did they choose? They've gone for degrees in divorce mediation. They've gotten jobs in weight-counseling programs or eating-disorder clinics. They work with psychologists as paraprofessionals; they take degrees in social work and assist abused children. These are native caretaker skills translated into gratifying, lucrative work.

Home-based businesses are perfect for any woman who by either choice or default is at home most of the day. This includes single women, too. Whether she is single or married, the home-based business is perfect for the woman with entrepreneurial skills who is not ready to open a shop or buy a business. She has the security of home, a place from which to launch what may turn into an extraordinary business five, ten, fifteen years down the line.

Let me give you an example. Your dream is to open a restaurant. You are a creative cook, but cannot invest the time or money in opening a business yet. How can you increase income and polish business skills? First, call businesses, friends, relatives. Describe your intention briefly—don't overdo or oversell. Tell them you are going into the catering business. Sound positive about it. See if you can make an arrangement with, for example, a beauty salon to bring in lunch for customers —nothing grand, just low cal and beautifully prepared. You need exposure. If the salon decides against food service, you might have connected with a number of working mothers under those driers who need your services to cook family dinners. Or put an ad in one of those ubiquitous penny-saver newspapers. Post notices on any bulletin board where there's a lot of traffic. Over 56 percent of mothers in America work or are looking for work. A percentage of those who do work live in your area, need your catering help and will be willing to pay for it.

There are a number of books on the shelf of any bookstore on the subject of home-based businesses, and they should give you an excellent picture of the qualities you need for success, as well as outlining how to go about building that business. Meanwhile, here are other ideas for you to think about.

- You are wonderful with children. You have a finished basement or large playroom that could accommodate eight children. There are a number of local mothers who need a loving, safe atmosphere for their children while they're at work. Enlist a friend in a similar situation and open a day care center.

- Your talent lies in clever footwork at the stores. You are a good shopper. Working mothers would appreciate your talents—they don't have the time to shop carefully and look for the best buys. While you are shopping for you, shop for them. Charge by the hour.

- You are perceptive about people and know how to get the best from them. Conduct seminars on how to hire a babysitter or how to train a sitter to be reliable and caring. Recruit sitters from local high schools and colleges and act as an agency, taking a percentage of the fee.

# Everyone Is a Contact

Contacts are people you know who know other people who can supply you with information about a job. If they can't, they may know someone with a line to a source. Everyone in your personal phone book who works or who has a working spouse is a contact. Any friend who doesn't work, but who can count a few relatives and friends in her personal phone book who *do* work, is a contact. Your butcher, your son's Sunday school teacher, your hairdresser are all contacts.

My assistant is a former client, a woman divorced after twenty-six years of marriage. She had never worked, but was ready to go out into the job market. "Can you type?" I queried. "With two fingers," she said dejectedly. "Learn how to type with four fingers and you've got a job." Why did I hire Iris? Charm, poise, intelligence, dazzling organizational skills perfected by being an admired hostess all those years—and a wonderful disposition. Who'd turn her down?

Men know the value of "networks," which is just another way of describing a connection to people who are usually in the same general business. When plum jobs are taken, it's often because the head of a company has kept a sharp eye out for talent elsewhere or knows whom to approach in his company to get a few names. You will most likely be starting at a low-level job. Even so, you can plug into networks. Find others who do what you want to do or can do. Tell everyone.

When we are young and think of the future, we transport the image of ourselves as we are now, not as we will be, into future time. At twenty, how difficult it is to imagine ourselves at forty-five or sixty. In our projected fantasy, we still have the strength and stamina of a young body, and the future holds more, not less. More youth, less age; more money, more fun, more travel, more family; less hardship, tears, disease. Understandable. But reality often brings us less.

Growing older is real, inevitable. It's no fantasy. But the future need not hold less or contain an excessive number of crises if we accept that a part of growing older is growing up. Work is one of the great assistants in that transformation from child to adult. Adulthood is a matter of coming to terms with who you really are and what *your* contributions will be to making your life a better one. When you are an adult, you can see a piece of yourself in others—the positive qualities as well as the disagreeable sides. Hopefully, this recognition will make you more compassionate toward others and toward yourself. When you are out there in the world, interacting with others who are not part of your immediate family, the experience enriches you. There is growth. And if you can get from these experiences a sense of humor about yourself and your life and not take it all so seriously, there's no reason that the future you dream of can't be yours. *You* need you to make it so.

Life is filled with pleasure and pain. Why not opt for more pleasure? Don't count on the future being brought to you on a platter by a man—there's always the possibility that your benefactor will change his mind, or maybe fate will do it for him. Your life can be better if you show some backbone. From it, you glean pride in your ability to contribute, care, give to yourself and by doing so, give to others. Productive work will do that for you.

# 8

---

# The Best Is Yet to Be

Today, this very day, you are the sum of all your days. Action, inaction, yeses, noes and maybes—they're all you. Perhaps history shows that you've lived with too many "shoulds," sliding too easily into accommodating others while neglecting yourself. The future need not hold restrictive patterns anymore—not if you're a smart cookie.

The future that lies ahead of you—the best that's yet to be—can be an exceptional one if you remember a few truths.

The first: The only person you will live your entire life with is yourself. This is not to say that the only person to live for is yourself, but that the only person you must rely on is *you*. Self-reliance or independence does not imply that you need no one else. Rather, as a self-reliant woman, you will understand that friends, husband, parents or children can leave to go on with their own lives. This creates both emotional and physical separations for all of you. But sadly, many women feel that when others depart, they are left with the short end of the stick—themselves! Smart cookies, though, are in touch with the greater part of who they are. They are not less, or inferior, or diminished when others choose to leave or if they choose to leave others.

They can be *more*. They have themselves and know how that counts.

The second truth: Smart cookies know that change is inevitable, that life holds crises, that dreams may fade but goals can be met. Self-reliant smart cookies can make new beginnings, not regret endings.

And the third: If you are still dreaming of a fair-haired prince to kiss you to wakefulness, or if you are waiting until opportunity singles you out and calls your name, you'll discover that as each year passes, you'll have little more than another birthday—no prince, no magical opportunity. Eventually, you'll just be a lot older and a lot sadder because there's less time for you to realize your goals and enjoy them.

*If your life is not to your liking, now is the time to take it off hold, make plans and move ahead.* You will be bringing new adventures, new experiences, new people into your world. These are the changes that make life richer. And, if there's any one idea I want to emphasize in this book, it's the *acceptance of change.* When you fiercely hold on to old dreams, your concept of a peak experience will be to brush your teeth with the tooth-brush of the man you love, or "breathe as he breathes." Five or ten years later your idea of a peak experience may be separate vacations. But that's okay. Why?

There will always be change—not only in relationships with others, but in how you feel about yourself, how your abilities can be developed, how learning can be varied and life-enhancing. Few of us can truthfully say that we will always feel one way or the other. Part of growing up—real maturity—is knowing that nothing stays the same and coping with that realization.

To change your life, you must first examine it carefully: What's right with it and what needs repair? Who's right for you, who's not? Can you honestly state that you could take care of yourself, with or without the pressure of economic need? Are you allowing yourself to grow, or are you adding to the burden of staying on hold by building upon excuses, rationales? To become an adult, to fully appreciate the pleasures of adulthood, you must take your life off hold. Change patterns one step at a time. Start goal-setting, figuring out what you need to make this life work for you.

When you get a sense of what your goals are and how to get there, others in your life may resist your efforts to expand, making it difficult for you to move ahead. What's on their mind? For one, they worry that if you are not who they need you to be—ready to serve or care for them while sacrificing your own goals and needs—they will be inconvenienced, challenged, and may even lose you. Too many women crumble under such pressures, especially from husbands and parents who demand that they be less than they, weaker than they. When others need you to feel inferior, they'll work long and hard to convince you they're right. They'll mock your goals, show little interest in what you want to do, insist you are a "little nothing."

Another truth here: Negative messages trap you within a limited life where you are ruled by others. *Tune out those messages* and you'll discover who you really are. You'll shake off that cloak of inferiority quickly enough. All it requires is positive messages that are self-created, self-directed, self-sustained and self-activated. You deserve success—whatever success means to you—peace of mind, having your needs met within a marriage, or finding satisfaction in a career.

The next significant course of action is mastering the

word NO. *No* is what keeps you from being taken advantage of by others. *No* is what stops you from working longer hours for no pay. *No* is what you say when your mother-in-law insists on joining you and your husband for a weekend in the country. *No* is what can keep you from getting pregnant when you don't have birth control. *No* is what gives you dignity. This one word, used wisely and well, can carry you through the day. You can refuse what you know in your heart is not in your best interest. *No,* said without rationalizations, excuses, or apologies, allows you to assert yourself.

*No* may create change, but many married women wait for their husbands to do the changing. They are afraid that if they change, their mates won't stand for it and will walk out. In many cases, neither they nor their husbands have grown during the marriage: the marriage has gone from "I do" to "I don't." Living together has become impossible, and the wife walks around resentful, shattered. What has happened? She has tied herself to Marriage, making it larger than life, larger than herself.

To go from "I do" to "I don't," and back to "I do," reposition that marriage, taking it from the exalted place above you and placing it shoulder to shoulder with your husband. Marriage is not a caste system in which you walk five steps behind a man or even three steps behind the children. *Widen the path; you are all equal.* Recognize that and you will have your second chance at making the marriage work with a foundation of respect, regard and caring. Marriage should make partners of you, not master and slave.

Should you want to terminate the marriage, you can do that and come to terms with that decision, too.

Make your decision without apology, regrets, or, much worse, lingering bitterness. Too many women remain divorced *to* their spouses, not *from* them, believing that the best part of their lives were spent in marriage, even if that marriage was a certifiably miserable one. With divorce, we feel that not only have we lost the man, but that he's somehow managed to take two lives with him—his and yours.

I hope you can prepare yourself to live without bitterness in divorce, to live with yourself knowing it's possible to love others. It may not be the same kind of love you experienced in your twenties, but that doesn't matter. When you are an adult, love can be better, richer, more compatible. Remarriage need not be based on sexual attraction, or on getting married because it's the thing to do.

Women who learn to deal with singlehood after divorce transform themselves into individuals more interesting to others and to themselves. They don't fret over who will take care of them now or in their old age. Though it will be natural to go through feelings of panic and desperation at the outset, know that there is a new life on the other side of those fears. As you live them through, it will become clear that by being true to yourself, you bring more to your life, not less.

A dear friend of mine was divorced ten years ago; Sally thought she wouldn't survive it. Of course, she did. She's recently moved out of the home she lived in for nearly thirty years—almost twenty of them with Verne—and into a building populated by single people about her age. She's organized exercise classes, bridge parties, dinners, and she's dating. Although Sally recognizes that she may meet a number of attractive men during the years that remain to her, she is being very careful about considering marriage, rather than acting rashly out of desperation.

In a way, Sally is a New Eve. She's gone through the transitions of being sexual and not sexual within marriage, being divorced, going through a brief period of promiscuity, and of occasionally choosing celibacy without feeling unsexed or undesirable as a woman. She can be close and intimate with a man without worrying if he'll make a commitment to her. She's been in love and wondered if marriage at that point would be right for her. Sally, the New Eve, does not live by sexual impulses. She knows there are choices to be made that would not have occurred to her twenty years ago. She can be affectionate to others, but sex need not grow out of that affection. She can sleep with a man and feel comfortable with it, awakening the next morning without the angst that arises, for some women, when there's no emotional commitment.

There's commitment of another sort that is as critical as selecting the man with whom you will share your life—commitment to work. Being a full-time homemaker is the highest-risk choice in careers that I can think of, a lot riskier than, say, being a typist who knows nothing about operating the computers her company is about to install. A homemaker's career ends just about when her children go off to school full time, or, if you like, when the kids get through college. What happens then? This woman is often in her mid-forties. She suddenly wonders how she will fill her time. Don't get caught in this trap! *Every woman owes it to herself to develop marketable skills.* The smart cookie goes through the homemaking years with an eye to growth, too, so she's not painted into a corner when it comes time for her to go out into the world. The clever woman knows she has one skill she's sure of and another in her back pocket. She looks ahead to see where the jobs will be, keeps up with the trends, finds ways to educate and train herself. Not only does work bring in money, it takes a woman out into the world, where there are relationships with others, friendships to be made, intellectual and emotional stimulation, and perhaps love.

There's a time when we give birth to children and a time to give birth to ideas. Our fifties, sixties and even seventies can be extraordinary years for us—the ages of entitlement. We can make our mark, see what's right (or wrong) with the world, and decide what needs to be done. Your twenties gave you a childhood, your thirties a true adolescence, your forties an adulthood. When you reach fifty, the age of entitlement lies ahead. You've paid your dues; you deserve some rewards. This can be a miraculous time, a time for coming to terms with your life, to explore, to achieve.

The age of entitlement need not be the so-called sunset years. Why wait for the light to dip under the horizon? Generate your own light and witness *that*. Know that there is no "later," only now. And if you think it's too late, give yourself the opportunity to prove this philosophy wrong. Inertia, bitterness, blaming, excuses—are all behind you during the age of entitlement. You have nothing to lose by going forward. If you set a goal and don't achieve it, there will be disappointment. That's okay. What matters is that you set your life in motion. If you missed one goal, set another. No one else can set your goals, bring you adventure.

*Will there always be a man in my life?* The question is frequently and urgently asked. The answer is maybe.

But there will always be *you* in your life. With you as the focus of this time you have on earth, you can complete unfinished business, examine relationships. There will always be those you love who don't love you back, don't approve of you. Don't be defeated by that. What's more important is that you approve of yourself, are comfortable in your own skin.

We all select what we want to be—for better or worse. During the age of entitlement, you are still in the process of becoming the best you can be, because the best *is* yet to be. You have a chance to live your life with integrity and grace. You deserve to be treated well—asking for benevolence or kindness from someone else is never as good as asking for it from yourself.

The age of entitlement ushers in maturity—and calm. The mature woman need not overreact, creating within herself tumultuous highs and lows. We learn by experience that good things don't happen instantaneously; it's a gradual process. There is no such thing as dropping ten pounds by Saturday night and keeping them off, or whispering the right words that will make a man fall desperately in love. During the age of entitlement we learn not to make long-term worries out of little issues and irritations. We are selective about whom we spend time with; it's not enough to just let others choose to spend your time. And time spent alone is pleasant, not desperate, isolated. By now, experience helps you to manipulate the world so things work harmoniously, productively.

I would like to leave you with a story of a woman who is both emotionally and physically sound—in fact, wonderful. Jean is a new friend, a vital, stylish, attractive woman much loved by many for her exceptional warmth, charm and wisdom. Jean has just turned sixty-five and looks, easily, fifteen years younger. We had a chatty lunch one day last summer, and decided on a stroll up Madison Avenue. Somehow the subject of relationships and how feelings can change within them came up. Jean stopped short, looked at me and said she wanted to confide in me a most remarkable experience.

When she was twenty-five, Jean was in love with a man three years younger than she. The relationship was an intense one. He was her first real love, her first lover. They planned on marrying, but his family exerted enormous influence on him—she was the wrong age, the wrong religion. He submitted to his father's wishes, and Jean broke up with him. She eventually married another man, had a child and built a successful career. Four decades passed. She did not know what happened to Tom.

While on a lecture tour in the South, she found out. A man in one of her audiences approached her after her speech to say that they had a friend in common— her first love. This go-between said that Tom would like to see her if she had the time. At the mention of his name, Jean felt herself flushing. It seemed impossible that she'd react so strongly to his name. She called him and they made plans for dinner. His wife would be joining them, too.

The night of the dinner, Jean was a wreck. Feeling like a love-struck teenager, she tore through the clothes she'd brought along with her, dissatisfied with every outfit. She chose one, dubiously, but settled on it. Did her hair look all right? Maybe it was too out of control—she should have had it cut. While putting on makeup, she stopped short as she peered into the mirror. Would Tom find her old and ugly? How much improvement could eye shadow make? And Tom? Would he be wizened and frail instead of strapping and tall? Finally she calmed down, reciting the facts to herself: She was sixty-five, sophisticated, mature, not a hysteric. She still loved her husband deeply and had a pleasant life with him. Why was this happening to her?

Then Tom buzzed from the hotel lobby; he'd be right up to get her. Heart pounding, she sat on the edge of the bed, hands in her lap, waiting for that fateful knock on the door. At last, Tom walked into the room. Jean told me it was as if forty years hadn't passed. Intense feelings for him flooded her; he was equally moved. He explained that his wife would meet them at the restaurant. Jean feared meeting the woman—what if Tom's wife were jealous? The more rational voice inside her coaxed her into control. Tom's wife appeared, a dimpled, pretty, effervescent, rotund middle-aged woman. Jean thought to herself, "Everything's okay and I look smashing."

At the end of the evening, Jean said goodbye to her old friend. She was shocked by her reaction to his parting kiss. She clung to Tom briefly. She felt her knees buckle and tears burn in her eyes. She couldn't believe it. She felt like a high-school girl leaving the boy of her dreams behind. Though she was married, Jean was re-experiencing love in its most breathless form.

Jean is not what I would call a glamorous woman: she is chic, appealing, and comfortable with her body. She has spent her life caring for others and helping them attain their goals. At sixty-five, when so many women think that their only profound feelings belong to what is lost and gone forever, Jean feels both for what *is* and for that which meant something to her in the past. She has earned the right to these feelings. She is entitled to them because she has cared for herself physically, professionally, and emotionally. She is a model for us all. She's alive!

The purpose of *Smart Cookies Don't Crumble* is to offer you a guide for getting on with your life. In order to do this there are three critical peaks you must conquer. The first is letting go of the past—forgive yourself for the errors of the past and take care of unfinished business so that you can move forward. The second is the affirmation of your worth. After all, in the words of the philosopher Hillel, "If you are not for yourself, who will be?" And the third peak is the recognition that you possess the power to give yourself the greatest gift in life—the adventure of your own life. Get on with it!